Intuitive Eating for Beginners

The Anti Diet Approach to Weight Loss and Disordered Eating

By

Monica E. Harris

INTUITIVE EATING FOR BEGINNERS
First Edition. July 29, 2020.
Copyright © 2020 Monica E. Harris

Disclaimer: The content in this book, Intuitive Eating for Beginners, is not intended to be a substitute for professional medical advice, diagnosis, or treatment. Always seek the advice of your physician or other qualified health provider with any questions you may have regarding a medical condition. Never disregard professional medical advice or delay in seeking it because of something you have read in this book. Reliance on any information found in this book is solely at your own risk.

The work contained herein has been produced with the intent to provide relevant knowledge and information on the topic on the topic described in the title for entertainment purposes only. While the author has gone to every extent to furnish up to date and true information, no claims can be made as to its accuracy or validity as the author has made no claims to be an expert on this topic. Notwithstanding, the reader is asked to do their own research and consult any subject matter experts they deem necessary to ensure the quality and accuracy of the material presented herein.

This statement is legally binding as deemed by the Committee of Publishers Association and the American Bar Association for the territory of the United States. Other jurisdictions may apply their own legal statutes. Any reproduction, transmission, or copying of this material contained in this work without the express written consent of the copyright holder shall be deemed as a copyright violation as per the current legislation in force on the date of publishing and the subsequent time thereafter. All additional works derived from this material may be claimed by the holder of this copyright.

The data, depictions, events, descriptions, and all other information forthwith are considered to be true, fair, and accurate unless the work is expressly described as a work of fiction. Regardless of the nature of this work, the Publisher is exempt from any responsibility of actions taken by the reader in conjunction with this work. The Publisher acknowledges that the reader acts of their own accord and releases the author and Publisher of any responsibility for the observance of tips, advice, counsel, strategies, and techniques that may be offered in this volume.

Table of Contents

INTRODUCTION 7

CHAPTER 1: WHAT IS INTUITIVE EATING? 9
- What Is Intuitive Eating? 9
- The History Of Intuitive Eating 10
- What are the Rules of Intuitive Eating? 10
- Intuitive Eating Rule #1. Adhere To Your Hunger 10
- Intuitive Eating Rule #2. Say No To The Diet Industry 11
- Intuitive Eating Rule #3. Don't Restrict What You Eat 12

CHAPTER 2: RE-FRAMING YOUR MIND 18
- Intuitive Eating Rule #4: Recognize When You Are Full 18
- Intuitive Eating Rule #5: Eliminate Dietary Thinking 19

CHAPTER 3: THE PITFALLS OF EMOTIONAL HUNGER 22
- What Is Emotional Hunger? 22
- Real Hunger Versus Emotional Hunger 23
- Intuitive Eating Rule #6. Don't Eat Out Of "Emotional Hunger." 23
- How To Determine Whether Your Hunger Is Emotional Hunger Or Actual Hunger 24
- How Food Cravings Often Indicate Emotional Deficiencies 26
- Examples Of Emotional Deficiencies 27
- How To Deal With Your Emotions Without Relying On Food 31
- How To Feel Your Emotions 35
- Intuitive Eating Rule #7. Listen to Your Body 36
- How To Eat When You Are Hungry 37
- How To Begin Listening To Your Body 38

CHAPTER 4: MAKING PEACE WITH YOUR BODY 42
- Intuitive Eating Rule #8. Don't Self Judge 42
- How To Make Peace With Your Body 44
- How To Get Away From Self-Judgement 46

CHAPTER 5: EXERCISE LIKE NEVER BEFORE 51
- Intuitive Eating Rule #9. Exercise Using Intuitive Movement 51

WHAT IS INTUITIVE MOVEMENT?	51
HOW CAN INTUITIVE MOVEMENT BENEFIT YOU?	51
SIMILARITIES AND DIFFERENCES BETWEEN INTUITIVE MOVEMENT AND OTHER TYPES OF MOVEMENT	53
HOW TO BEGIN USING INTUITIVE MOVEMENT	56
CHAPTER 6: MINDFUL EATING	**61**
WHAT IS MINDFULNESS?	61
HOW CAN MINDFULNESS BENEFIT YOU?	61
HOW TO BEGIN USING MINDFULNESS IN YOUR LIFE	62
WHAT IS MINDFUL EATING?	66
HOW CAN MINDFUL EATING BENEFIT YOU?	67
STEPS TOWARDS THE PRACTICE OF MINDFUL EATING	69
HOW TO PRACTICE MINDFUL EATING	71
CHAPTER 7: INTUITIVE EATING MEAL PLANNING	**73**
WHAT IS MEAL PLANNING?	73
HOW DOES MEAL PLANNING DIFFER WITH INTUITIVE EATING VERSUS DIETING?	74
HOW TO MEAL PLAN WITH INTUITIVE EATING	74
CHAPTER 8: INTUITIVE EATING RECIPES	**76**
INTUITIVE EATING RECIPE EXAMPLES	76
Delicious Coconut Date Smoothie	*76*
Egg And Avocado Rice Bowl	*78*
Breakfast Oats	*81*
Braised Chicken On A Bed Of Lentils And Mushrooms	*82*
Beef And Broccoli Stir-Fry	*84*
INTUITIVE EATING WITH FOOD ALLERGIES OR RESTRICTIONS	86
TIPS FOR INTUITIVE EATING WITH FOOD ALLERGIES OR RESTRICTIONS	86
INTUITIVE EATING RECIPES FOR FOOD ALLERGIES OR RESTRICTIONS	87
Fresh Green Beans with Tofu And Mushroom Stir-Fry	*87*
Vegan Chana Masala Curry	*89*
CHAPTER 9: INTUITIVE EATING WHILE PREGNANT	**91**
CRAVING EXAMPLES AND SUBSTITUTIONS	91
FOODS TO AVOID	92
INTUITIVE EATING POST-PREGNANCY	95
CAFFEINE POST-PREGNANCY	95
BONUS: HOW TO TEACH YOUR CHILD MINDFUL EATING	**97**
HOW TO TRANSFORM YOUR CHILD'S RELATIONSHIP WITH FOOD	97

How To Encourage Your Child To Practice Intuitive Eating 98
How To Encourage Your Child To Practice Mindful Eating 98
Intuitive Eating Quick Tips 101

CONCLUSION 103

Introduction

For many years, I struggled with binge eating and found myself bouncing from diet to diet with little results. Like most women, I spent countless hours worried about my body image, all the while struggling to control my weight. Through the ups and downs, I found myself resorting to disordered eating, which didn't help my situation. In fact, it made it worse.

I felt stuck. Hopeless at the idea of ever being able to kick the habit and lose weight.

Chances are, you might relate to this feeling. You might be finding yourself at a crossroads with your weight, health or dieting in general. Worse yet, if you are like me, you may have found yourself having a rocky relationship with food.

If you are frustrated with dieting and unable to stop disordered eating, this book is written for you!

When I learned about the non-diet method of intuitive eating, a major shift occurred in my life. I saw diet culture as the enemy and found that my own connection to my body allowed me to open my eyes about how I ate. Over time, my thinking changed radically and my health improved as a result. This method has been proven to work for many people with different body types. And after reading this book, you can be one of those people too.

Intuitively eating is not a quick fix or a fad diet. It's a lifestyle and mindset that will benefit many aspects of your health. By following this non-diet method of intuitive eating, you will find numerous benefits including the following:

- Higher self-esteem
- Better body image
- More optimism
- Lower body mass indexes
- Higher HDL cholesterol levels
- Lower Triglyceride levels
- Lower rates of emotional eating
- Lower rates of disordered eating

According to scientists who published an article in the Journal of the Academy of Nutrition and Dietetics, this method of eating is proven to help people lose weight for good, and to maintain their healthy weight once they reach it. Also, this "non-diet" approach led to improvements in cholesterol levels.

Through reading this book, you will be sure to develop new perspectives on dieting and eating, along with new perspectives on exercise. You will also find new ways of looking at your body and the importance of loving yourself. This will ultimately lead you to gain a new lease on life. There has never been a better time to take your eating habits and your lifestyle into your own hands and change it for the better.

If you want to start feeling and living more optimally, the information in this book will help you do so.

This book will allow you to find a solution for your weight and eating struggles. I guarantee that it will exceed your expectations in terms of how it will change your mind forever. You will thank yourself for choosing this book as you move forward in your life.

Get ready to start your journey in the next chapter, where we will begin by looking at the theory of intuitive eating and how it can help change your life for the better.

Chapter 1: What is Intuitive Eating?

Let us start by looking at what exactly intuitive eating is, as well as a brief history of how this style of eating came about. This chapter will provide you with a solid foundation of knowledge on which to build your new lifestyle.

What Is Intuitive Eating?

Intuitive eating, at its core, is a style of eating that puts you in the driver's seat of your own life. The practice of intuitive eating encourages you to listen to your body. This, in turn, allows you to provide your body the foods it needs *when it needs them.*

Intuitive eating is different than a traditional diet. Instead of following a set of guidelines that tell you when and what to eat, you learn to listen to your body because it has all the answers.

Intuitive eating does not limit certain foods or require you to stick to restrictive meals exclusively, but instead encourages you to learn as much as you can about what your body is telling you in regards to its hunger and needs.

There are two main components to intuitive eating:

- Eat when you are hungry
- Stop eating when you are satiated

As odd as it may seem, humans are very far from this kind of eating in today's world. With so many diet trends and numerous "rules" for how you should and should not eat, it can be difficult to put these ideas aside and let your body do the talking.

The History Of Intuitive Eating

Though it may seem as though intuitive eating is a concept that has been around forever, it is a relatively new concept as far as modern eating styles go. The origins of intuitive eating are said to be dated to around 1978 when a book called "Fat is a Feminist Issue." was written. This book discussed many of the same types of ideas around eating, diet culture, and body image.

Similarly, in 1995, two women wrote a book about intuitive eating, which aimed to help women to achieve a better body image and experience less guilt around eating. This is when the term "Intuitive Eating" was first developed, and it has been used to describe this style of eating ever since.

While the beginnings of intuitive eating are rooted in feminism and the pressure that is put on women by diet culture, both men and women can benefit from it. It is a style of eating and living that is best for the human body in general.

What are the Rules of Intuitive Eating?

In this section, we are going to look at the foundational rules of intuitive eating. I will begin by explaining what these are, and then we will examine the best approach to take when it comes to making a change in your life, especially when this change is related to the way that you eat.

These rules serve to outline the philosophy of intuitive eating and how it can be employed in anybody's life. Over the next several chapters, we will look at many of these concepts and how they can help you gain a better understanding of intuitive eating.

Intuitive Eating Rule #1. Adhere To Your Hunger

In diet culture, hunger is seen as an enemy. However, when it comes to intuitive eating, hunger is not an enemy, but rather a source of valuable information for you regarding what your body is asking for and what it needs.

The main philosophy behind rule number one is: You must respect your hunger.

This means that you must respond when your body signals the need for nutrients and sustenance. If you don't acknowledge your hunger, you will likely wait until you are ravenous before eating. If this is the case, you will be much more likely to overeat. If instead you had trusted your hunger and eaten when you first became hungry, you would have eaten the right amount and been much less inclined to overeat. When you choose to adhere to your hunger and eat when your body tells you that it needs sustenance, you are much more likely to eat just the right amount, and you and your body will be satisfied rather than completely stuffed afterward.

You must reject feeling shameful and angry for being hungry and learn to feel happy that your body is telling you what it needs. Be thankful that you can provide it with nutrients for it to keep working hard for you!

Intuitive Eating Rule #2. Say No To The Diet Industry

At first glance, the diet industry may seem like it is concerned with helping people to improve their lives. However, this is not the case. In reality, the diet industry is concerned with making money.

The diet industry grows their revenue by convincing people that they should try a specific diet plan, followed by, another and another. People who fail to find results when following these diet plans will try many different diet trends, spending large amounts of money in the hopes of finding one that finally works.

The diet industry is also focused on making you feel like you are not perfect enough. Looking at your body from the perspective that it is not perfect will ultimately leave you feeling like a failure. Since you will never achieve perfection, you will never feel satisfaction from these diets. For this reason, you will forever be chasing the "right diet" when, in fact, there is no "right diet," there is only the best way that you can fuel your own personal body by giving it what it needs. This is where intuitive eating comes in.

When it comes to being healthy and taking good care of your body, intuitive eating is not a diet. It is instead a philosophy that aims to help you return to the traditional way that humans ate before diets were created.

To follow intuitive eating properly, you must acknowledge that the diet industry itself is harmful to you. You must begin to embrace that your own body holds the key to effectively losing weight.

Intuitive Eating Rule #3. Don't Restrict What You Eat

When trying to make a lifestyle change or trying to modify habits that are firmly ingrained in your day to day life, the approach you take will play a large part in whether you succeed or relapse. The basics of this principle will pave the way for you to start taking real action and start taking steps toward a new way of eating that will improve your life. This principle is all about not falling prey to restrictive eating.

Intuitive eating is a good choice for anyone, especially for those who prefer more flexibility when it comes to their eating time and those who do not want to restrict their meals at all. Humans should not be putting themselves through boot camp every time they feel hungry, and this method does not adhere to that type of mindset.

One of the reasons that intuitive eating is such a successful and cherished form of eating is that it allows the body to lead the mind in the right direction when it comes to seeking out its needs.

Paying attention to the messages your brain is sending your body and knowing how to deal with them is essential. For example, did you know that your cravings could be giving you much more information than you give them credit for? Below we will look at what your cravings could mean and why you should let your body guide your eating choices.

A craving is an intense longing for something (in this case food), that comes about strong and sudden.

In your case, that longing is probably for a certain food. When we have cravings for specific foods, it can mean more than what it seems. While you may chalk it up to simply being hungry, your cravings may instead be indicating a nutrient deficiency.

Why is this? A craving comes about because the body thinks that the nutrients it needs can be gained through eating a certain food. As a result, the body tells you that it wants that particular food. This is why a craving feels so urgent. The body is trying to help itself by telling you what to eat. But to us, this feels like an intense craving.

Sometimes the things we crave won't be the best way to get the vitamins or minerals that we need. Having the nutrients that you need in the right amount helps to regulate mood, hunger, and cravings. Thus, when one or more of these nutrients are low, it is hard for us to regulate our appetite and our cravings, and this is why we tend to long for foods that are not always the best ways to receive these nutrients. For this reason, understanding your cravings can help you give your body exactly what it needs.

- Chocolate And Magnesium

When we crave chocolate, this means our body is low in Magnesium. Dark chocolate naturally contains high levels of Magnesium.

When you are experiencing a craving for chocolate, it usually comes in the form of a craving for a doughnut or a chocolate bar. The problem with this, is that this form of chocolate contains high amounts of sugar, fat, and oil, and not enough magnesium to help your body combat this craving for good.

The next time you crave chocolate, keep in mind that it may be due to a magnesium deficiency. Other signs of a magnesium deficiency can include general sugar cravings, which explains why you crave sweets.

When your body consumes sugar, it must use magnesium in order to process it for digestion. For this reason, giving in to your cravings of sugar may actually end up further reducing your body's magnesium levels, which will send you into a cycle of more sugar cravings and an increasing level of magnesium deficiency.

Chocolate by itself is actually quite rich in nutrients. However, it is the actual pure cocoa that holds all of these nutrients. If you are going to eat chocolate to ease your sugar cravings and your need for magnesium, make sure that it is dark chocolate. To get the most nutrients possible, be sure that the dark chocolate you choose comes with at least 70% cocoa content. Cocoa contains high levels of magnesium, iron, fiber, and antioxidants. While you are getting your magnesium fix, you will also be getting your fill of other good nutrients that your body needs.

If you have low magnesium levels, there are many other ways you can replenish it. Eating nuts like almonds and cashews is a great choice as they are high in magnesium and may give your body exactly what it needs. If you crave chocolate, try eating these magnesium-rich foods at your next meal and your chocolate craving may just dissipate.

- Hydration

If you are craving juice or pop or other sugary drinks, consider that you might be dehydrated and, therefore, thirsty. Sometimes we see drinks in our fridge, and since we are thirsty, we want to reach for them. Sometimes, however, we are simply in need of water. After all, water is the best thing to quench your thirst.

The next time you are craving a sugary drink, try having a glass of water first, then wait a few minutes and see if you are still craving that Coca-Cola. You may not want it anymore once your thirst has been quenched.

- Salty Foods

If you are craving salty foods like chips or pizza, your body might be low in Sodium. We must be careful with this one as being low in sodium is quite rare given our modern diets. It could be, however, if you sweat a lot that this deficiency occurs. If this is the case, though, try reaching for something more natural like celery, milk, or even beets. While these may seem like odd sources of sodium as they don't taste particularly salty, these three foods contain natural sodium. They are also not nearly as bad for the body as fast foods are.

- Meat

If you are craving meat, you may feel like you want some fried chicken or a hot dog. This can indicate a deficit of iron or protein. The best sources of protein are chicken breast cooked in the oven, while iron is best received from spinach, oysters, or lentils. If you think you may not like these foods, there are many different ways to prepare them, and you can likely find a way that you enjoy. As long as they are not fried, this will be much better for you than a hot dog or fried chicken. The other way to get iron is from lean beef, which can be found in a lean steak.

Craving meat can also mean that you are lacking in vitamin b12. Vitamin B12 is found in meat and other animal products. Vitamin b12 helps the body to have a healthy bloodstream as well as a good memory. To get this, you want to eat good sources of organic meats as well as eggs and turkey.

- Calcium

If you find yourself craving cheese, it could be because of a Calcium deficit. To find out if this is the case, you need to try eating other foods that are rich in calcium and see if your craving dissipates. Calcium-rich foods include tofu or leafy green vegetables like kale, spinach, or arugula. Some forms of cheese contain good amounts of calcium and do not include additives and preservatives. Examples of these include mozzarella and feta cheese.

- Fatty Foods

If you find yourself craving fatty, carbohydrate-dense foods like muffins or high-fat baked goods, you could have an omega-3 deficiency. Omega-3 is a type of fatty acid, which is usually found in oils or fats. These specific types of fatty acids are called "essential fatty acids" because the interesting thing about omega 3, is that our bodies actually cannot produce it. This is what makes it essential, which means that we must ingest it for our bodies to have any at all. Because of this, you might see many people take Omega-3 supplements, or you may find eggs sold in the grocery store that have omega-3 written on the packaging.

So, if this is the case, what foods should you be eating to get this essential nutrient? Omega-3 can be found in the following food sources:

- Fish such as salmon and tuna

- Nuts and seeds like walnuts, flax seeds, or chia seeds- the types of seeds that you would add to smoothies or smoothie bowls.

Adding the foods listed above into your diet can help you to get this essential nutrient. By learning more about common cravings and what they could be telling you, you can begin to learn more about your body. This will help you to listen and observe what it is telling you, so that you are not restricting your diet and, in turn, keeping your body deprived of something it needs.

Chapter 2: Re-Framing Your Mind

In this chapter, we will examine intuitive eating rules #4 and #5 and look at how these ideas will come into play in your new lifestyle. These rules are critical in outling how you should think when adopting the intuitive eating lifestyle.

Intuitive Eating Rule #4: Recognize When You Are Full

It can be hard to determine how much you should eat or when you have had enough without eating to the point of feeling stuffed.

Many times, we keep eating until we are full, sometimes to the point of making ourselves feel physically ill. We want to avoid this, as the goal anytime you eat is to give your body what it needs so that it can function optimally for you. In this section, you are going to learn how to take care of your body, because stuffing it to complete fullness is not what it is asking for.

There are a few different ways that you can deal with this. Using these techniques, you can help yourself realize when you are satiated. Keep in mind, it will take some time to train your mind to understand when you have eaten enough. With enough practice, you will be able to recognize the signs of satiety much earlier. Below are a few ways you can begin recognizing when you are full.

1. Pay close attention to your body as you are eating. When you feel like you may be satiated, stop eating and wait for about twenty minutes. You will likely feel full then, but if not, you can always eat a bit more after the 20 minutes passes.

2. Before you eat, drink a glass of water. This will help you to eat just the right amount and not too much, as this will allow you to have something in your stomach already when

you begin eating. This will also help with your digestion as the water will allow everything to move smoothly along your digestive tract.

3. Another way to recognize when you are full is by eating more slowly. When we eat, it takes about twenty minutes for the hormone in our bodies that tells us that we are full to reach our brain. Our stomach signals to our brain that we are hungry, and that signal takes about twenty minutes to actually reach the brain. Thus, we want to make sure that we eat slowly so that we can precisely tell when we are full. If we eat very quickly, by the time we get the signal that we are full, we will have already eaten much more than we may have needed.

Intuitive Eating Rule #5: Eliminate Dietary Thinking

This rule will help you turn your mind away from dietary thinking and towards a newer, more productive way of viewing your relationship with food and hunger.

If you force yourself to change like a drill sergeant in an aggressive manner, you will end up being unnecessarily tough on yourself every day. The result will be feelings of failure and defeat.

Forcing yourself to do anything in life will not lead to long-lasting change. You will eventually become fed up with all of the rules you have placed on yourself, and you will be inclined to abandon the goal altogether.

If you approach change with rigidity, you will not allow yourself time or space to look back on your achievements and congratulate yourself. Thus, you may fall off of your plan into an even more extreme and unhealthy lifestyle than you had before. You may end up having a week-long binge and falling into worse habits of eating. To further illustrate this concept, I have outlined something called *The Deprivation Trap* below.

The Deprivation Trap is something that can occur when you approach dieting with a strict mindset. What this means is that you become stuck in something called a *thinking trap*. When this occurs, you become focused on what you can't have and what you are restricting yourself of, instead of what you *can* have. You become hyper-focused on everything you aren't allowing yourself to have. You then become resentful of the fact that you aren't able to just eat whatever you want.

After a while, because you are focusing so intently on what you can't have and the fact that you can't have it, you decide that you are just going to have it anyway. This decision comes from a feeling of anger and entitlement. The next thing you know, you have gone on a binge, and after restricting yourself completely for some time, you have now undone any progress you made in a single sitting.

You will then begin to feel terrible about yourself and what you have done, and will feel the need to punish yourself. Thus begins the cycle of deprivation.

It is quite difficult to avoid this trap when you are trying to make lifestyle changes through food deprivation. It is quite rare that a person, no matter how strong their willpower, will be able to completely deprive themselves of something without first easing themselves off of it. A sudden and strict deprivation is not natural to our brains and will leave us feeling confused and frustrated.

Instead of approaching your diet and eating habits with this kind of dietary thinking, intuitive eating encourages you to instead listen to what your body is telling you. By using your body as the guide for your personal eating schedule and plan, you will not fall into the deprivation trap.

Instead of following a diet plan that another person made for you, you will make your own rules. Nobody else knows your body as well as you do, so why let them tell you what you should and should not eat? Instead, listen from the inside, and that will be the only guide you need when it comes to eating.

Chapter 3: The Pitfalls of Emotional Hunger

This chapter contains a wealth of information about emotional hunger and emotional eating, as well as many strategies and tips for how you can conquer it. We will discuss the Intuitive Eating Rule #6 and define the term *Emotional Eating* for you to help you to understand it.

Also in this chapter, you will find information about emotional eating and how it affects your brain and your body. We'll cover some reasons why people emotionally eat and how to tell the difference between actual hunger and emotional hunger.

What Is Emotional Hunger?

First, let us begin by defining the term *emotional hunger*. This section will help you to determine whether this is something you suffer from.

Emotional hunger or emotional eating occurs when a person is suffering from emotional deficiencies of some sort. This includes lack of affection, lack of connection, or other factors like stress, depression, anxiety and general feelings of sadness or anger.

Therefore, to reduce the negative feelings they are experiencing or to feel better about them, they will find comfort through ingesting food. This is called emotional eating.

Some people turn to this type of eating on occasion, such as during a breakup or after a bad fight with someone. When this occurs several times in a week for a prolonged period, this type of eating can negatively impact a person's life. Over time, it can become a never-ending cycle of hopelessness that leads to bigger problems.

Real Hunger Versus Emotional Hunger

Sometimes it can be hard to tell when we are really hungry, and when we may be feeling as though food will make us feel better emotionally.

Real hunger is when our body needs nutrients or energy and is letting us know that we should replenish our it soon. This happens when it has been a few hours since our last meal, like when we wake up in the morning, or after a lot of strenuous activity such as a long hike. Our body uses hunger as a signal that it requires energy and that if it doesn't get it soon, it will begin to use stored energy sources as fuel. While there is nothing wrong with the body using its stored fuel, this signal is a sign that we should eat to replenish those energy stores.

Perceived hunger or emotional hunger is when a person thinks they are hungry, but their body doesn't require any more energy. This could happen for several reasons:

1. The brain notices that it is the time of day when you would normally eat, even if we have just eaten a short time before.
2. You are feeling stressed or anxious, and your body isn't sure of how to soothe this so it thinks that food may help.
3. When your emotional state makes you crave comfort and positive feelings, knowing that you can obtain these from certain foods.

Intuitive Eating Rule #6. Don't Eat Out Of "Emotional Hunger."

Emotional hunger occurs because eating foods that we enjoy makes us feel rewarded on a biological and chemical level within the brain. If you are wondering why a person would continue to eat emotionally when this is known to cause problems in their life, it is because the sense of reward that they feel encourages them to eat more. This intense feeling outweighs the possibility of future negative consequences as a result of eating too much.

How To Determine Whether Your Hunger Is Emotional Hunger Or Actual Hunger

In this section, we will look at the different types of hunger and how you can tell them apart. This will help you to distinguish when you are hungry and when you may be turning to food to soothe your emotional state.

When we feel hungry, there are several questions we can ask ourselves to determine which category we fall into. Below, I have listed the questions to ask and what they can tell us about our hunger.

1. *When did I last have a meal?*

You should ask yourself this question because if you had a full meal less than 2 or 3 hours ago, it is likely that you are not experiencing actual hunger. Still, the hunger is coming from something else like an emotional need or boredom.

2. *How hungry am I?*

Go within and ask yourself how hungry you are. While you don't want to wait until you are starving and light-headed to eat, you want to be hungry enough to warrant eating. If you are not quite at a level where you could eat a meal, you probably aren't hungry enough to eat just yet.

3. *Am I still hungry now?*

If you feel hungry, try drinking a glass of water. Wait twenty minutes and see if you are still hungry afterward. If you are not, you could have just been hungry because of your emotional state.

4. Was there a change in my emotional state previously?

Sometimes, we will feel the need or the compulsion to eat right after we get some bad news or have an upsetting thought or conversation. Ask yourself if you felt the feeling of hunger directly after one of these occurrences or something that you know to be a trigger for your emotional hunger. If something like this has just happened, you may not have connected them as being related. By taking a minute to recognize this, you can decide that you may not actually be hungry and address the emotional issue instead.

5. Do I feel hungry again right after eating?

If we begin to eat or have a snack when we feel emotional hunger, you may feel good right afterward, but shortly after, it will not be resolved. This is another way to find out whether you are actually hungry or not. If you do decide to eat something and shortly after feel hungry again, you were likely not hungry for food but had an emotional need instead. Since this emotional need could not be resolved with food, you feel hungry and crave that positive feeling you get right after eating.

6. Do I feel guilty about eating?

If you eat when you are hungry, you will feel satisfied and ready to continue with your day. You will not feel any sense of guilt or shame about it because you were simply fueling your body. However, if you ate when you had a craving and you felt hunger, but it was an emotional need telling you that you were hungry, you may feel guilty or ashamed afterward about having eaten.

This feeling can indicate that you were not hungry but that you were trying to fill a void that was not filled by eating food.

The reason that hunger doesn't become improved or disappear after eating is that the body craves food for that positive feeling that we get after we eat. Eating certain foods or craving the addictive chemicals within the food, makes us feel rewarded and happy temporarily because of the reaction in our brain that is similar to taking a drug. Our mind enjoys this feeling, and it helps to lift our mood or take our mind off of our emotional turmoil for the moment.

The problem is that when these rewarding and positive feelings are gone, we return to feeling the way we did beforehand. The only way to truly resolve our emotions or feel better about something is to face them head-on. Trying to solve them by other means like eating or distracting ourselves will only work in the short term and will leave us feeling those same negative emotions after the distraction is gone.

In the next section, we are going to look at how you can begin to deal with your emotions in healthy and productive ways, without using food as a means of coping.

How Food Cravings Often Indicate Emotional Deficiencies

To assist you in your practice of dealing with your emotions safely, I will share some of the most common emotional deficiencies that people face. These emotional deficienies are the causes that lead people to seek out food as a means of coping. First, though, we will look at one of the most prominent theories behind this and how the study of emotional hunger is helping people who suffer from it to make beneficial changes in their lives.

While other types of cravings can occur (such as the cravings that pregnant women experience, or those that indicate nutrient deficiencies), there are some strategies that you can use to determine whether your cravings are being caused by a true emotional deficiency. This begins by examining which exactly foods you crave and when they crave them.

For example, if you feel like eating a pizza every time you experience high levels of stress, or if you are depressed and you begin eating a lot of chocolate, this could indicate emotional eating.

Conversely, if you crave fruits like a slice of watermelon on a hot day, you are likely just dehydrated, and your body is trying to get water from a water-filled fruit that it knows will make it more hydrated. This is an example of a regular craving that indicates your body is simply seeking water in the form of fruit. On the other hand, if you often feel hungry when you are at home, and you live in a house full of turmoil and frustration, this could indicate emotional hunger.

Examining things and situations like this leads scientists and psychiatrists to explore this concept in more depth and determine what types of emotional deficiencies can manifest themselves through food cravings.

Examples Of Emotional Deficiencies

There are several types of emotional deficiencies that can be indicated by hunger. We will explore these in more detail, in hopes that you will recognize some of the reasons why you may be experiencing disordered eating.

- Childhood Causes

If you think back on your childhood, think about how your relationship with food began. Maybe you were taught that when you behaved, you received food as a reward. Maybe when you were feeling down, you were given food to cheer you up. Maybe you turned to food when you were experiencing something negative. Any of these experiences could lead someone to suffer from emotional eating in adulthood. This tumultuous relationship with food was something you may have learned early on.

This type of disordered eating is quite difficult to break as it has likely been a habit for many years. When we are children, we learn habits without knowing, and we often carry these habits into our adult lives. While this is no fault of yours, recognizing it as a potential issue is important to make changes.

- Covering Up Emotions

Another emotional deficiency that can manifest itself in emotional eating and food cravings is the effort to cover up our feelings. Sometimes we would rather distract ourselves and blanket our emotions than to face them head-on.

In this case, our brain may make us feel hungry to distract us from the emotions we are experiencing. When we have a quiet minute where these feelings or thoughts would pop into our minds, we can cover them up by deciding to prepare food and eat. We convince ourselves that we are "too busy" to acknowledge our feelings because we have to deal with our hunger.

The fact that it is hunger that arises in this scenario makes it very difficult to ignore and very easy to deem as a necessary distraction since, after all, we do need to eat to survive. This can become a problem, however, if your body does not require nourishment.

If there is an issue in your life that you think you may be avoiding or if you tend to be very uncomfortable with feelings of unrest, you may be experiencing this type of emotional eating.

- Feeling Empty Or Bored

When we feel bored, we often decide to eat or convince ourselves that we are hungry. This occupies both our mind and our time, while making us feel less bored, sometimes to the point of feeling positive or happy.

We can also eat when we are feeling emotionally empty. This void can be a general feeling of dissatisfaction with life, or the feeling of lacking something important.

When we feel this way, the food will quite literally be ingested to fill the void. This will inevitably lead to an unhealthy cycle of trying to administer our emotions with something that will never actually work. We will become disappointed every time and continue trying to fill this void with material things like food or shopping.

Examining the true reason behind the void is difficult, but will help you greatly in the long term. Being able to recognize when hunger is masking another issue is key to ending disordered eating for good. Doing so will also help you to identify ways to fill the emotional void that can be more healthy and productive, such as group fitness or taking up a new hobby.

- Affection Deficiency

Another emotional deficiency that could manifest itself as food cravings is an affection deficiency. This type of deficiency can be feelings of loneliness, feelings of a lack of love, or feelings of being undesired. If a person has recently gone through a breakup, or if a person has not experienced physical intimacy in quite some time, they may be experiencing an affection deficiency.

This type of emotional deficiency will often manifest itself in food cravings as we will try to gain feelings of comfort and positivity from the good tasting, drug-like foods that have allure us.

- Low Self-Esteem

Another emotional deficiency that may be indicated by food cravings is a low level of self-esteem. Low self-esteem can cause people to feel down, unlovable, inadequate, and overall negative and sad. This can make a person feel like eating enjoyable foods will make them feel better, even if only for a few moments.

Low self-esteem is an emotional deficiency that is difficult to deal with, as it affects every area of a person's life. This includes their love life, social life and career. Sometimes, people have reported feeling like food was always there for them when nobody else was. While this is true, they will often be left feeling more empty and down on themselves after giving into cravings.

- Mood

A general low mood can cause emotional eating. While we all have general low moods or bad days, if this makes you crave food multiple times per week, this could become emotional eating.

- Depression

Suffering from depression also can lead to emotional eating. Depression is having a continuous low mood for months on end which can cause a person to turn to food for comfort and a lift in spirits. This, in turn, becomes emotional eating.

- Anxiety

Having anxiety can lead to emotional eating, as well. Both general anxiety (constant levels of anxiety) and situational anxiety (triggered by a situation or scenario) can lead to emotional eating.

You have likely heard of the term *comfort food* to describe certain foods and dishes. The reason for this is because they are usually foods that are rich in carbohydrates, fats, and are generally heavy. These foods bring people a sense of comfort and are often turned to by people suffering from anxiety, because they help to provide temporary relief. These foods make them feel calmer and more at ease. However, this only lasts for a short time and their anxiety usually gears up again.

- Stress

Stress eating is probably the most common form of emotional eating. While constantly being on the go, stress is increasingly more common in today's world. While this does not become an issue for everyone experiencing stress, it is a problem for those who consistently turn to food to ease their stress. Some people are always overwhelmed, and they will constantly be looking for ways to ease this feeling.

Food is one of the ways that people make themselves feel better and take their minds off of their stress. As with all of the other examples we have seen above, this is not a lasting resolution, and it becomes a cycle. Similar to the cycle of emotional eating that we discussed, the same can be said for stress. Unlike emotional eating, stress eating can make you feel more tense, as you feel like you have done something you shouldn't have, which causes you to become more frazzled. Thus, the cycle ensues.

There are many different emotional causes for the cravings we experience. A person's emotional eating experience is unique and personal to them.

You may find that you experience a combination of the emotional deficiencies just mentioned. Many of these can overlap, such as anxiety and depression, which are often seen together in a single person. Whatever your struggles are, know that there is hope for recovery. This is what the rest of this book is designed to help you with, as it will allow you to reframe your relationship with food.

How To Deal With Your Emotions Without Relying On Food

As you can see from what we have discussed so far, recognizing the struggles you face involving food will help you to recover from being a person who uses food as a coping mechanism. This will help you to move towards being a person who has a healthy relationship with eating and become someone who can deal with their emotions in healthier ways.

Recognizing the things with which you struggle will help you to figure out how to deal with them. Nobody can force anybody else to make a change, especially an entire lifestyle change. So, recognizing the struggles that you are facing will allow you to be in charge of your journey to recovery.

Recognizing the food-related struggles you face will also help you to have a better relationship with your body. Instead of viewing your body as something that you dislike, you can begin to love it and care for it. You can do this by providing it with nourishment, clean energy, and adequate hydration. Viewing your body as something to care for as it carries you around all day will allow you to shift your view of yourself and see your body in a more positive light. You will begin to view it as something that you work together with instead of something that you work against.

Recognizing your struggles will also help you to have a better relationship with your mind. Understanding how your mind works will help you to better take care of it. You will be able to recognize your feelings and what they could be caused by, and then treat them in a way that will help it to feel better.

Bettering your relationship with food and your relationship with your body will also improve your relationship with your mind. This is because you will begin to provide it with what it needs. Which will, in turn, lead to better cognitive functioning, control over impulses and decision-making.

Doing some serious and deep self-reflection is not an easy process but a necessary one when it comes to healing yourself and changing your ingrained habits. Looking deep within and asking yourself the right questions will help you to take the first step.

The first step is to acknowledge your issues and find the sources of them. Finding the sources will tell you exactly what you need to face and deal with to find lasting change in the form of this new intuitive eating lifestyle.

If changing your life is done as a distraction from the underlying issues, the change will not be lasting. These issues will rise to the surface again eventually, and they will manifest themselves in strong cravings. I want you to be able to change your life permanently, and to do this we will begin with some deep self-reflection. This step is the most crucial and perhaps the most difficult. Try to keep your mind focused on the life you want because it can be yours. You deserve happiness and health! You will get out of this workbook what you put in, so take your time as you go through this chapter and try to get in touch with the deeper parts of yourself.

We will begin the self-reflection with some questions that you can ask yourself to get into a self-examination mindset. Complete this workbook, and you will be well on your way to dealing with your emotions.

The first question you will ask yourself is a rather obvious one, but this will make it easy for you to get a start on your self-examination.

1. Do I feel like I struggle with emotional eating?
Yes ____ No ____

2. Do I wish to find out the underlying causes of my emotional eating?
Yes ____ No ____

3. Do I feel like it is time for a lifestyle change in terms of my eating habits?
Yes ____ No ____

4. Have I been diagnosed with any mood-related disorders (such as depression, bipolar disorder, or anxiety)?
Yes ____ No ____

If your answer is yes, you skip the next set of questions. If you answered No, or you are unsure, answer the following:

5. Do I have long periods of low mood or an anxious state?
Yes ____ No ____

6. Have I been feeling this way for the last 3 to 6 months?
Yes ____ No ____

7. Do I often feel disconnected from my life?
Yes ____ No ____

8. Do I often feel nervous and worried about worst-case scenarios?
Yes ____ No ____

9. Do I often catastrophize in my head when thinking about things that are to come?
Yes ____ No ____

10. Do I often feel drastic swings between very high moods (like happy, excited and motivated) and very low moods (sad, down, hopeless)
Yes ____ No ____

If you answered mostly Yes to the 6 questions above, you might suffer from a mood-related disorder. While this questionnaire is not conclusive and is not sanctioned by a doctor or a medical professional, this could give you a bit of direction when it comes to your mood, your emotions, and the causes of your emotional eating. I encourage you to dig deeper if you feel like a question resonates with you. Positive change will come out of finding and addressing the root of your problem.

Knowing that the cause could be something like depression, anxiety, or other mood disorders can help to give you some clarity about your mental state. If you think this could be the case, consider visiting your doctor (or someone knowledgable in these areas) to talk about this further.

How To Feel Your Emotions

It is very important to notice and address your feelings, as they can have many important things to tell you.

Pay attention to your thoughts. Whenever you feel a negative emotion, work backwards. Try to figure out what thoughts were just on your mind before you felt negative emotions. Emotions that you should be looking out for are stress, anxiety, self-loathing, sadness, demotivation, anger, and frustration. These emotions are the ones that typically cause a person to choose instant gratification.

Just like how you will be paying attention to the thoughts that occurred before feeling a negative emotion, pay attention to the thoughts that occurred before feeling a positive one. Typically, when a person is feeling positive emotions, it creates more motivation and inspiration to reach goals.

One great way to begin feeling through your emotions is by self-reflecting on them and noticing when they are causing your struggles with food. Recognizing your triggers is important because this will help you to understand the differences between feeling emotional hunger and feeling actual hunger.

What are some triggers related to your emotions or specific emotions that make you seek comfort in the form of food? Are there any triggers that you experience that cause your emotional deficiencies to flare up? For example, you may think the following:

- "When I feel scared, I begin to crave sweets."
- "When I am lonely, I want a cookie."
- "When I get stressed, I want a salty snack."

If you become hungry, you can look back on your day or the last hour and determine if any of your triggers were present. If they were, then you will be able to determine that you are likely experiencing emotional hunger, and you can take the appropriate steps instead of giving in to the cravings blindly.

When you experience a trigger that causes one of your emotional deficiencies to come to the surface, this will be a time that you will most likely to turn to food as a means of comfort and as a way to self-soothe. Recognizing what these triggers are will help you to recognize when to intervene in your thought process.

Instead of giving into cravings after an emotion triggers your feelings of loneliness, you will intervene and say to yourself, "A trigger just occurred, so I am going to call a friend and talk instead of eating what I crave."

Intuitive Eating Rule #7. Listen to Your Body

The seventh intuitive eating rule is one that is very important when it comes to intuitive eating, and it is arguably the most important of them all.

Intuitive eating comes down to listening to your body, so this list would not be complete without rule #7. While it may seem obvious to some, to many other people, listening to your body is quite a difficult thing to do. In a society where there are so many distractions, something seemingly as simple as listening to your inner self can be quite a difficult task. In this section, we are going to look at some tips for listening to your body and how this will benefit you when it comes to emotional eating.

How To Eat When You Are Hungry

When we discussed emotional eating in the previous section of this chapter, we looked at a list of questions that you can ask yourself when determining whether you are genuinely hungry or if you are experiencing emotional hunger.

If you ask yourself all of the above questions, and you determine that you are experiencing actual hunger, the next step is to take action and nourish your body with healthy and delicious foods.

While some people determine that they are experiencing actual hunger, a problem arises though when they subsequently begin to feel a series of self-judgments and second guesses. These can be thoughts like the following:

- Should I eat?
- Do I deserve to eat?
- Am I going to eat or am I going to wait?

When you live according to the intuitive eating mindset, you are not going to enter this spiral of thoughts, but you will instead feed your body.

The key to intuitive eating is to eat when you are hungry, but not when you are ravenous. If you are only mildly hungry, you can likely stand to wait a little bit to eat. As a rule of thumb, when you start to become mildly hungry, begin to prepare your meal so that by the time you finish, you are at the perfect level of hunger as you sit down to eat. If we wait to eat until we are ravenous, we will have let our blood sugar drop to quite a low level and we will likely have begun to get light-headed, irritable, and have difficulty with decision making. If you feel like this when you are beginning to eat, you will want to make a note to eat a bit earlier next time.

How To Begin Listening To Your Body

If you are experiencing a flurry of negative emotions when you decide that it is time to eat, you will be focused on your emotional state rather than on tasting and enjoying the food that you are eating.

While we have touched on this briefly in the book already, the reason that emotional hunger can become such a problem for so many people is that your body learns over time that eating certain foods (such as those containing processed sugars or salts like fast food and quick pastries), makes it feel rewarded even though the end result is often guilt.

When you are sad or worried, your body feels negative and looks for ways to remedy this. Your brain then decides that eating those fast foods will make its emotional state more positive. As a result of this process, (which happens entirely in the background of your mind), you will consciously feel a craving for those foods. These foods usually include sugary snacks or salty fast-food meals, and you may not even be aware of why you crave them.

If you decide to give in to this craving and eat something like a microwave pizza snack, your body will feel rewarded and happy for a brief period, which reinforces to your brain that craving food to make itself feel better has worked. If you end up feeling down and guilty that you ate something that was unhealthy, your brain will again try to remedy these negative emotions by craving food, and a cycle of emotional eating will begin.

Emotional hunger and listening to your body go hand in hand, which is why they have been included in the same chapter of this book. By understanding your emotions and what they mean, you will make room to listen to your body without having to find an unhealthy way to distract yourself from uncomfortable feelings.

Listening to your body includes both mental and physical signs that your body is sending to you. We have already talked about emotional or mental signs, so now we are going to talk about the physical signs.

One of the best ways to begin listening to your body is by doing meditation, or by being mindful. We are going to talk about something called *mindful eating* later on in the book, but for now, we are going to focus on using mindfulness as a means of getting in touch with your physical body.

The Body Scan Practice is a technique that can be performed multiple times a day to help you identify what you are feeling physically and mentally. Using this technique, you can learn to release the stress carried in your body and mind. Most of the time, when you are stressed, it's very common for it to be held in different areas of your body in the form of tense shoulders, stomach pains, or side aches. A lot of the time, you likely aren't even aware of the stress that you are carrying in your body. During periods of extra stress, you may be feeling a lot of physical discomfort but not necessarily connect it with your emotions.

The body scan meditation method is effective in relieving stress not only from the mental aspect but in the physical aspect, as well. Research points to the fact that there are numerous physical and psychological benefits to relieving tension and relaxing your body. Relieving physical tension has been proven to lower psychological stress even when you aren't using any external stress relief efforts for the mind. Relieving tension in your body can decrease overall lower levels of stress, which then leads to less physical tension. This meditation works to break the vicious cycle of mental and physical tension that feed off each other. Due to this, the body scan meditation is a very effective and useful meditation technique that allows you to remain both physically and mentally relaxed. ("Body

Scan Meditation", 2019). It can help you return to a calm state when you notice that you've become too tense. Here is how to perform body scan meditation.

1. Find a comfortable place where you can sit down and fully relax your body. It's easier if you are lying down, but sitting down is effective as well. Try to find a position that is comfortable for you but not so comfortable that you may fall asleep easily. Bring awareness to your breath. Let it slow down and start breathing from deep within your belly instead of your chest. Let your abdomen expand and then contract with each breath you take. If you find your shoulders moving up and down while breathing, bring your attention to your belly and allow the breathing from there. Pretend as if it's a balloon inflating and deflating your abdomen as you take each breath.

2. This is where we begin to do the actual 'body scan.' Pretend that there is a scanner above you (if you are lying down) or in front of you (if you are sitting down). Imagine that this scanner expels a laser beam that is slowly scanning your body. It begins at the top of your head. Bring your awareness to where that scanner is and slowly move it down your body. Do you notice any tension that you feel as you move the scanner through your body? Do you feel any tightness on your shoulders, neck, back, or stomach? Do you feel any sensations of pain, whether it's subtle or sharp? Are you feeling any areas of concentrated energy in your body? If you notice and feel something that is off, try to acknowledge it and think about why it might be. If there is tension, release it and move on. Continue to scan your body all the way from your scalp to your ears, cheeks, chin and neck. This becomes more automatic and much easier with

practice to the point that you will be able to do this very quickly and with less effort.

3. Make sure you're bringing attention to areas that you've discovered that have uncomfortable sensations. Breathe into them and watch what happens. Try to imagine the tension leaving your body through the exhale of your breath. A lot of people notice that the tight feeling becomes more intense at first, but continuing to meditate through the discomfort allows it to dissipate. Keep your awareness focused on that feeling for a few moments; make sure you are staying present. Feel free to give yourself a light massage in that area if it helps and move on to the next part of your body when you're ready.

4. Continue to do this scan with each area of your body, moving from your head to your toes. Make a note of how you feel and which body parts are holding stress. Helping release tension in your body now will allow you to be more aware of it in the future so you can relieve it as you feel those sensations.

Try to practice the body scan meditation several times throughout the day or during times where you feel stressed. If you are short on time, you can do an abbreviated version of this meditation by sitting down and bringing awareness to any place in your body where you feel tension.

Chapter 4: Making Peace With Your Body

In this chapter, we are going to learn about the importance of making peace with your body and how you can begin to do this. We are first going to look at the eighth rule of intuitive eating and how this relates to coming to terms with your body.

Intuitive Eating Rule #8. Don't Self Judge

This rule is very difficult for many people.

You cannot fully embrace the practice of intuitive eating if you have nagging feelings of self-judgment each time you take a bite of food or decide that you are going to eat lunch when you are hungry. In this section, we are going to look at some strategies for dealing with and overcoming self-judgment.

Let us examine this intuitive eating rule with an example. Let's say you are trying to focus on healthy eating, and you find that you have had trouble doing so. Maybe you ate a cupcake, or maybe you had a soda at breakfast. From the perspective of a traditional diet mentality, this would pose a problem for the diet, and this can lead to feelings of regret and disgust. You would likely be beating yourself up and feeling terrible about the choice you have made.

It is very important to avoid beating yourself up or self-judging for falling off the wagon. This may happen sometimes. What we need to do is focus not on the fact that it has happened, but on how you are going to deal with it and react to it.

There are a variety of reactions that a person may have to this type of situation. We will now examine the five most common reactions and their characteristics.

1. The person may feel as though their progress is ruined and that they might as well begin another time again, so they go back to their old ways and may not try again for some time. This could happen many times over as they will fall off each time and then decide that they might as well give up this time and try again, but each time it ends the same.

2. The person could fall off of their diet plan and tell themselves that this day is a write-off and that they will begin the next day again. The problem with this method is that continuing the rest of the day as you would have before you decided to make a change will make it so that the next day is like beginning all over again, and it will be very hard to begin again. They may be able to begin the next day again, and it could be fine, but they must be able to heavily motivate themselves if they are to do this. Knowing that you have fallen off before makes it so that you may feel down on yourself and feel as though you can't do it, so beginning again the next day is very important.

3. Similar to the previous case, the person may fall off, but instead of deciding that the day is a write-off, they tell themselves that the entire week is a write-off, and they then decide that they will pick it up again the next week. This will be even harder than starting the next day again. Multiple days of eating whatever you like will make it very hard to go back to making the healthy choices again afterward.

4. After eating something that they wish they hadn't, that wasn't a healthy choice, they will decide not to eat anything for the rest of the day. This is done to avoid eating too many calories or too much sugar. It may be the easy choice to decide that the next day they will begin again. This is very difficult on the body as you are going to be quite hungry when bedtime rolls around. Instead of forgiving yourself, you are punishing yourself, and it will make it very hard not to reach for chips late at night when you are starving and feeling down.

5. This reaction is the best for success and will make it much more likely that you will succeed long-term. If you fall off at lunch, let's say, because you are tired and in a rush, and you grab something from a fast-food restaurant instead of going home for lunch, there is a way to deal with it. First off, you will likely feel like you have failed and may feel quite down about having made an unhealthy choice. Instead of starving for the rest of the day or eating only lettuce for dinner, you will put this slip up at lunch behind you, and you will continue your day as if it never happened. You will eat a healthy dinner as you planned, and you will continue with the plan. You will not wait until tomorrow to begin again; you will continue as you would if you had made that healthy choice at lunch. The key to staying on track is being able to bounce back. The people who can bounce back mentally are the ones who will be most likely to succeed. Without question, you will need to maintain a positive mental state. This will help you to look forward to the rest of your day and the rest of your week in just the same way that you were before you had a slip-up. One bad meal out of the entire week is not going to ruin all of your progress and recovering from emotional eating is largely a mental game. It is more about mindset than anything else, so we must never underestimate the role that our thinking plays in our success or failure.

How To Make Peace With Your Body

Self-care is one of the best ways to begin making peace with your body. There are numerous ways that you can practice self-care, and they can be different for everyone. In this section, I will outline some ways that you can practice self-care to begin feeling more positive about yourself and your body and begin changing your internal environment.

- You Are Worthy

This is a great exercise to use to remind yourself of everything that you love and appreciate about yourself and your life. Take time to write down all of the things that you love about yourself and your life. This will remind you of all of the positivity surrounding you and will serve to uplift you.

- Limit Negative Influences

By limiting the negative influences in your life, you are making a statement to yourself. You are showing yourself that you place importance on preserving your mental health. When you remove negative influences and limit your exposure to things or people that make you feel negative, you are prioritizing yourself. This is a great way to practice self-care and can give you a sense of worth.

- Support System

Finding a positive and uplifting support system helps improve and preserve your mental health. This can be one person or a group of people. Your support system can include family, friends, or acquaintances, as long as they support you in your journey and help you to feel positive about yourself. Some examples of places that you can find a support system include Facebook groups, support groups, weight loss support groups and book support groups. Not only will a support system help you to move toward positivity, but when you begin to make changes in your life, your support system will help by supporting you in maintaining these changes.

- Journaling

Another exercise that you can do to change your mindset is to write down all of the limiting beliefs you think you possess. Next, try to write down where you believe they came from. For example, consider where you may have learned to think in this way. Having this information written down in front of you can help you to begin reforming your inner beliefs, as awareness is the first step to change.

How To Get Away From Self-Judgement

Self-judgement is something that everybody deals with to some degree. In this section, we are going to look at how you can take back the reins when it comes to your thoughts and feelings about yourself and how you can begin to shift them.

- Be aware

Awareness is the first step that needs to be taken to recognize your inner-critic and to reshape it into something less critical and more supportive. Try to pay attention the next time you are feeling distracted, tense, or anxious. Try to identify whose voice is the voice of your inner critic. Try to find the situation where this voice awakens. It allows yourself to dig deep and identify the most vulnerable feelings during situations where your inner critic is awake. These feelings or these situations are likely what your inner critic is trying to protect you from feeling. However, by protecting you, they are holding you back from meeting your full potential.

When people have developed unhelpful thinking processes, it is hard to make decisions to benefit their future self because their thoughts create negative emotions that drive away motivation. Some people argue that by simply increasing your willpower, thus overcoming the need for instant gratification, you will be able to fix your situation. This belief, however, is not an effective solution for long-lasting change. In this section, we are going to look at a variety of ways that you can begin to combat those limiting beliefs and the negative self-talk that goes on in your mind.

- Remind Yourself To Be Positive

As we learned, bad habits are built through many years, and no amount of willpower can handle overcoming that many bad habits in a person's life. Rewiring your brain to minimize the amount of negativity you feel in the first place is a much more efficient method to approach this problem.

- Catch Yourself Thinking According To Your Limiting Beliefs

Often, if the person had just paid attention to their thought process, they would be able to catch themselves before their mind automatically spiraled to a place of complete de-motivation. By catching yourself before you get there, you can prevent yourself from falling into your negative thought patterns that are limiting you and holding you back.

- Show Yourself Evidence Against Your Limiting Belief

Showing yourself evidence that supports or doesn't support the thoughts that are on your mind will help you to change your limiting beliefs. By showing yourself evidence, you can cancel out those negative thinking styles and give yourself the confidence and motivation to overcome any situation.

Often, people who are stuck in a mindset of, "I'm going to fail and embarrass myself anyway, so why bother?" will choose to not prepare. This leads to a feeling of failure when they inevitably do not achieve success. This further solidifies their limiting belief.

When your inner critic begins to tell you that you can't do a certain thing, or you're not good enough, or you're not worthy enough, simply find evidence within your past life experiences that challenge or discount this belief. Prove your inner critic wrong and show them why holding you back is only going to do more harm than if you failed whatever task you were planning to do. The more you tell your inner critic this, the more they will learn to listen to you and help you in another way that is not just preventing you from doing things.

- Ask For Support From Your Inner Critic

If your inner-critic is telling you that you are going to embarrass yourself, you can prove it wrong. You can do this by using evidence-based arguments and then asking for its support by saying "This is a difficult challenge for me, and I want to overcome it. I need you to support me, regardless of the outcome."

Remember, your inner critic is just another version of yourself. Be kind to it even if it's not being kind to you. Showing yourself, kindness is very important in our case.

- Negotiate With Your Limiting Beliefs To Change Them

When you notice these voices and statements that are going on in your brain which are related to your limiting beliefs, you can then simply acknowledge them and begin to negotiate with your inner critic. Let them know that you thank them for looking out for you, but you are confident in your ability to make decisions for yourself. You can let them know that even though you may fail and feel embarrassed, it is still better than a lifetime of holding yourself back. Since your inner critic is a part of you, it can listen to reason as long as you allow yourself to be reasoned with.

- Surround Yourself With Positive People

Surrounding yourself with people that can encourage you and foster positivity will also change your inner-critic's opinion. Often, hearing positive compliments from other people holds heavier weight in your mind when compared to you telling yourself the same thing. Try spending time with people who are supportive of your goals and the changes that you are looking to make in your life. It will make your journey a little bit easier.

Limiting beliefs and negative self-talk, as well as negative body-image, can lead a person to feel terrible about themselves, often to the point of feeling like they hate themselves. As I mentioned earlier, to make lasting changes, we are going to work on loving oneself instead of hating oneself. By seeing your body in a positive light, appreciating it for all of the things it allows you to do, you will begin to make choices with the health of your body in mind. This will lead to lasting, positive changes for your physical and mental health.

- Be Gentle with Yourself

It is important to be gentle with ourselves because we are usually our own toughest examiner. We look at ourselves very critically and we often think that nothing we do is good enough. We must be gentle with ourselves so as not to discourage ourselves. We must not put ourselves down, or make ourselves feel bad about what we are working so hard to accomplish. We must remind ourselves that everything in life is a process and does not happen instantly, and we mustn't tell ourselves to "hurry up and succeed," as we often do.

When you fall off track, you must not beat yourself up for this. It is important to be gentle with yourself. Beating yourself up will only cause you to turn into a spiral of negativity and continue to talk down to yourself. This will make you lose motivation and will make you feel like you are a failure. Having this state of mind will make it difficult not to turn to food for comfort.

You must avoid this entire process by avoiding beating yourself up in the first place. If you don't beat yourself up and instead encourage yourself, instead of thinking that it is too hard and then turning to food for comfort, you will not feel the need to find comfort at all. Instead, you will talk to yourself positively and encourage yourself from within. Then, instead of making yourself feel bad, you will instead make yourself feel motivated. You will be ready to continue on your journey.

Even if you don't fall off of the plan, it is still important to talk to yourself nicely and with encouragement. You must recognize that changing your behaviors that are ingrained in your life is no small feat. You must encourage yourself just like you would encourage someone else. Think of it as if you were talking to a good friend of a family member who was going through this instead of you. What would you say to them? How would you say it? You would likely be quite gentle and loving in your words. You would likely tell them that they were doing a great job and to keep it up. This is exactly how you want to speak to yourself from within and the exact types of words and phrases that you want to use. If we spoke to our friends the way we speak to ourselves most of the time, they would be quite hurt. Thus, we must remember this when trying to motivate ourselves, and we must be gentle.

Another way to be gentle with yourself is to avoid being too restrictive in the beginning. You must understand that it will be a challenge, and easing into this new lifestyle will be best. Beginning by making small changes and then adding more and more changes as you go will be a good way for your mind and body to get used to the changes. If you dump a lot of changes on yourself too quickly, this will feel like a burden for both your mind and body.

Chapter 5: Exercise Like Never Before

In this chapter, we are going to look at our final intuitive eating rule, and then we will spend some time discussing the importance of exercise and how it relates to intuitive eating.

Intuitive Eating Rule #9. Exercise Using Intuitive Movement

The ninth and final intuitive eating rule does not involve eating, but instead involves movement. Movement is an important part of overall health and wellbeing, which is why it is included in this list of rules. We will begin by looking at what intuitive movement is, and then I will share with you how you can begin making it a part of your life.

What Is Intuitive Movement?

Intuitive movement is the practice of moving according to the needs and wishes of your body. It can be viewed in the same way as intuitive eating, except with the movement of your body instead.

How Can Intuitive Movement Benefit You?

Exercise is great for our body, mind, and overall health. Adding an exercise regime into your life is as important, if not more, than any other measures you take to maintain your health. Exercise has been proven to help with a variety of things in life such as stress, impotence, and cellular repair. As you know, all of our body systems work together to form the person that we are. If one of them isn't functioning quite as well as it should be, all of the other systems feel it too. Exercise works on all of these systems at the same time, and if one of them isn't firing on all cylinders, exercise will help that system to wake up, improve, and stay healthy.

Exercising will show you what your body can do and how strong it is, which in turn will make you feel stronger mentally. Exercising will help you take your mind off of those nagging cravings and will give you more clarity overall. You are then able to look deep inside at those cravings and the emotional issues that are causing them. Exercise will help in all aspects of your life and will help you to continue reaching for recovery.

For any level of exercise, challenging your body in new ways will be beneficial in so many aspects of your life. In addition to its effects on the brain, body, and mood, it will help with your health in the long-run and the ease with which you will be able to complete everyday tasks like climbing the stairs or throwing a ball to your child. The goal is to make this a part of the new lifestyle you are working towards, which will make it so ingrained in your life that you will not want to be without it.

There are also chemical benefits to exercising that will assist both your body and mind. When we exercise, our brain releases chemicals that tell us we enjoy the effects that the exercise is giving us. This feeling is known as "runner's high," and it is that elation you feel after you run a long-distance or complete a workout.

When you are feeling sad, and you exercise, your mood will lift because of this runner's high. For this reason, it is not important what kind of physical exercise you do, but rather the fact that you simply engage in exercise period. Doing this regularly will help you feel motivated and will keep your mood positive.

This feeling of *runner's high* can be compared to the rewarded feelings that high-sugar foods give us. The difference is that with runner's high, the feelings of elation and accomplishment last way longer than the rewarded feelings we get from eating food.

Fast food makes our brains feel happy, but our body feels heavy and lethargic. Exercise, as I mentioned, makes your body feel great, and this is why the effects of runner's high are so long-lasting.

Similarities And Differences Between Intuitive Movement And Other Types Of Movement

Many people begin following some type of exercise plan to get in shape or to lose weight. Sometimes, this does not lead to success. People often end up having to try to force themselves to perform exercise that doesn't feel good for their body, that has not been personalized for them, and which they find no enjoyment in. This often lasts for a week or two, after which the person becomes fed up and decides that having to push themselves to perform the exercise plan is not worth the potential benefits.

On the other hand, intuitive movement involves a deeper motivation and an enjoyment factor that is not often present in other kinds of exercise regimes. If you enjoy the movement, you are much more likely to want to perform it, and you will not even need to force your body to do it, as you will genuinely want to take part in it.

As I mentioned earlier in this chapter, I am going to show you how all of the rules of intuitive eating can be applied to intuitive movement. Here, I will break down each one of them and show you how this kind of intuitive mindset can be applied to many different areas of your life to give you a new way of viewing yourself.

- *Intuitive Eating Rule #1. Adhere to Your Hunger*

This first rule is related to hunger and eating in particular, but if we instead change it to "Adhere to your body's wishes" in terms of movement, this can be understood to mean that we must listen to and follow our body's desires when it comes to movement and exercise.

- *Intuitive Eating Rule #2. Say No to The Diet Industry*

The diet industry often involves an exercise component that is rooted in the same basic principles as the diet plans that are trendy today. For example, if you are on a no carbohydrate diet, this often comes with the expectation that you will exercise in a certain way for a certain number of days in the week. By saying no to the diet industry, you are also saying no to boot camp-style exercise that you must force your body to do.

- *Intuitive Eating Rule #3. Don't Restrict What You Eat*

This intuitive movement principle is another important one. Don't restrict what you eat, and don't restrict how you move. For example, if you find joy in going for a long walk, don't restrict your movement by thinking that that is not an acceptable form of movement. When it comes to intuitive movement, anything goes, as long as it makes your body feel good!

- *Intuitive Eating Rule #4. Recognize When You Are Full*

Recognizing when you are full is important for intuitive eating, as well as recognizing when you are finished exercising. To avoid injury, pay attention to what your body is telling you and recognize when it has felt the benefits of your movement and when it is time to take a rest. Resting is an important part of intuitive movement.

- *Intuitive Eating Rule#5. Eliminate Dietary Thinking*

Eliminating dietary thinking, as well as eliminating the "boot camp" thinking when it comes to exercise, are both important. Instead of forcing yourself to attend a workout class that you hate or making yourself eat celery every day of the week, listen to your body and allow it to guide your movements.

- *Intuitive Eating Rule #6. Don't Eat Out of "Emotional Hunger."*

Emotional hunger is a concept that is quite specific to food, but it can also be applied to movement. If you are feeling negative emotions or if you are feeling down, you likely do not feel like moving your body at all, let alone partaking in some sort of exercise. When this happens, it is important to listen to your body and find out what will make it feel good in a healthy way. For example, you may wish to binge on a bag of chips in times of stress, but instead try to find something healthier to help you feel better. Exercise is a natural stress-reliever and anti-depressant. Maybe you wish to take a walk and get fresh air, or maybe you wish to leisurely swim in the pool. Whatever your body is telling you, follow that instead of trying to force yourself to do something that you will hate.

- *Intuitive Eating Rule #7. Listen to Your Body*

The number one principle of intuitive movement is to listen to your body. Your body knows what it wants and what it needs, so you must learn to trust this and listen to it. Over time you will get better at this, but for now, you will need to keep reminding yourself to do so, especially when it comes to exercise and movement.

- *Intuitive Eating Rule #8. Don't Self Judge*

Self-judging is something that everyone must deal with, and it can be quite a challenge to silence those voices in the back of your mind that are telling you all kinds of judgmental things. Instead of thinking, "I should be going to the gym right now," try to think positively about the movement that you have done or try to remember that your body needs rest, and if that is what it is asking for, then give it rest.

- *Intuitive Eating Rule #9. Exercise Using Intuitive Movement*

Exercising using intuitive movement is something that you will need to learn how to do, and it will likely involve a lot of unlearning as well. The first step is to learn to be gentle and kind with yourself and learn how to listen to your body and what it is telling you its needs are.

How To Begin Using Intuitive Movement

In this section, we are going to look at how you can begin using intuitive movement in your own life. Whether you are a seasoned runner or someone who has never exercised before in your life, there is an exercise routine out there for you that your body will enjoy. I will begin by sharing some different types of exercises that you can do. If you do not have much experience with exercise, you can begin to explore different types of movement to find out what your body enjoys the most.

Cardiovascular exercise and resistance training are two different types of exercise that people can benefit from. Cardiovascular exercise is the type of exercise that involves an elevated heart rate due to activities such as running, riding a bicycle, or swimming. This type of exercise is often referred to as "cardio." It is a type of exercise usually done for an extended period at a steady state.

Resistance training is a type of exercise that involves using weighs to build up your muscles by doing things like squats, push-ups, bicep curls, and so on. This is the type of exercise that you would often do if you go to a gym to exercise. Contrary to popular belief, this type of exercise will not make you bulky and muscular, especially if you are a woman. Instead, it will give you more tone and a leaner body.

When we engage in cardiovascular exercise, our heart rate increases, what this does is carry more oxygen to our muscles so that they can keep exercising. It also carries more oxygen to our brain. More oxygen and blood flow to the brain means that your brain will work more efficiently, more sharply, and with more clarity after you finish exercising. More blood flow to the brain also means that it will be generally healthier.

Exercising often and for a continuous period helps to keep the brain healthy and in working order. This helps with memory, decision making, and learning.

Exercise is also the most effective antidepressant. Many pills are prescribed to treat and beat depression, but the most effective and natural way of boosting your mood (and keeping it up) is through exercise.

When we exercise, we become stronger, faster, and more agile. This not only helps us to exercise better but it helps us in our everyday lives. Moving through life with more ease than before is a great feeling that can only be achieved through physical exertion. Our bodies are built to move, and they love it when we do! Our bodies are made to continually grow stronger the more we do, and this is what inevitably happens as soon as we begin exercising consistently. You will also begin to see aesthetic changes as well. You can see your muscles growing, your body toning, and your fat disappearing. These changes on the inside and the outside make us feel great about the body we live in, and about the progress we are making.

Taking the time to exercise and to stick with an exercise regime of any sort, as long as it makes your body and mind feel good, shows our body that we are willing to do the hard work that exercising takes, and it also shows our mind the same thing.

Do not be discouraged by your experience level when it comes to exercise, as everyone can benefit from it, and everyone must start somewhere. Below, I have given you several ideas for exercise, no matter the experience level you bring with you.

If you normally don't do much exercise or much walking around, begin by taking the stairs. Start by deciding to walk when you go to certain places, like to the store down the street or to a friend's house. Audiobooks and music can be a way of taking your mind off of what you are doing and make exercise more enjoyable. Beginning with this type of movement will get your body used to moving again and will get your muscles and joints working smoothly.

If you occasionally walk, like to the bus stop or the store on your lunch break, you can begin with a little bit more exercise than someone who is sedentary. Since your muscles and joints are likely somewhat used to being in a standing position, you can begin to jog a little bit. You can also jog after dinner around the block a few times, or jog to the store and walk back every few days. You could also take a yoga class if you wish or do some video-guided yoga at home.

On the other hand, you may already have a moderate level of walking included in your life and occasionally speed that up to a jog. If this is the case, you can begin to move your body around in new and different ways. Try doing some sit-ups and push-ups at home before or after your run. Alternatively, run to the neighborhood park and use the playground equipment to do some chin-ups, some jumps onto a step, or some running up and down the stairs. This will keep your heart rate up and teach your body new ways of moving while allowing your upper body muscles to get a bit of attention.

If you run frequently and you benefit from some bodyweight exercises now and again, try visiting a gym. At the gym, try doing some exercises with weights. You can try squatting, pressing some things overhead, and maybe some bicep curls. This will challenge your muscles in ways that your body weight cannot and take you to a new level of fitness and mood-boosting.

Finally, if you are an experienced runner, you are likely quite familiar with the feeling of runner's high. You are likely quite familiar with how exercise can change your mood around and take you from feeling hopeless to hopeful. If you want to try some new forms of exercise, try adding a gym routine using small weights. This will take your running to new heights and will give you a new type of exercise experience to break up the running days.

Continue to challenge yourself in new ways and teach your body new ways of moving. Exercise does nothing but good things, so keep up your routine.

There are some things to note if you are a woman. Since exercising helps women to regain some of the muscle mass lost with increasing age, it can be greatly beneficial for women to exercise into their older years. It is important to be aware of how to do this safely, though. It can be safer to stick to low-impact exercises, so avoid exercises that include jumping or any sort of quick, jarring movements. Instead, spending some time on an exercise bike (or a real bike) or an elliptical machine can be good as they both reduce impact and are therefore better for a woman's joints. Things like running involve more impact, so if you have joint pain, it is best to avoid this type of exercise. Further, lifting small weights or walking with weights in your hands can help you to build back some muscle. This will lead to an increase in your resting rate of metabolism. This is the number of calories your body burns when it is just sitting at rest to do things such as breathing or sitting. Your overall health will be greatly improved by an increase in muscle, the improvement of your joint health, and the lowered risk of diseases such as heart disease (which can be reduced by doing aerobic exercise).

If you are a person who hates running or traditional exercise, that is okay too! Luckily, there are numerous other exercises that do not fit into either of the two categories. These include exercises such as yoga, Pilates, high-intensity interval training and group training classes. While these are not considered to be traditional methods of exercise, they are no less valid than resistance training or cardiovascular exercise. Many people who are not too enthused about exercise wish to pursue methods that incorporate more of a social aspect or those that are slower in their movements. If this is what you prefer, this is just as valid as going for a run! There are even more ways to be active such as pursuing activities like gardening, dancing, hiking and kayaking. Any activity that raises your heart rate and brings you a sense of joy can be used as an exercise in combination with a diet change to provide you the health you are looking for.

Exercise meets you where you are, and your brain will gladly take any form of the new movement as a mood booster. When you enjoy the exercises that you are taking part in, you are much more likely to choose to engage in them more often and much less likely to find excuses to avoid them. By enjoying what you are doing, it will feel like a reward and not like a punishment. For this reason, be sure to choose a form of exercise that you enjoy.

The important thing here is that you are moving intuitively and that this is leading you to feel better in the body that you are in. Additionally, it should help you to realize that your body is an amazing vessel that allows you to do so many incredible and enjoyable things!

Chapter 6: Mindful Eating

In this chapter, we are going to look at mindfulness as it relates to eating. I will begin by defining mindfulness for you before moving onto something called mindful eating. This chapter will help you to learn how to be present in your life without distraction, which will lead to lifestyle improvement and a better relationship with food.

What Is Mindfulness?

Before we jump in, let's first learn about the basics of mindfulness. Mindfulness is most popularly achieved through the use of meditation. In modern society, psychology professionals describe meditation as a way to achieve mindfulness. It can be described as a method of focusing one's thoughts, and mind on an activity or object to train their awareness and attention. The goal of this is to help the person achieve clear-headedness and an emotionally calm, stable state. You may think that mindfulness sounds easy, but it is a very difficult activity to master.

Mindfulness is something that requires strong self-discipline. Simply just listening to a mindfulness podcast or going to one meditation class isn't going to help you become a mindful person.

How Can Mindfulness Benefit You?

The most popular reason that people decide to learn meditation is actually to achieve mindfulness to combat mental obstacles. If you are someone that lives a very fast-paced and stressful life, mindfulness and meditation can help you manage your thoughts and emotions to bring you more peace. Many doctors who specialize in the area of mental health have begun to study and even practice meditation and mindfulness techniques to promote a healthier brain and mind. Others take the practice of meditation and mindfulness to another level and aim to reach a high level of spirituality. When an individual can achieve mindfulness, they can increase their overall life satisfaction.

How To Begin Using Mindfulness In Your Life

You can practice mindfulness while washing the dishes, and nobody would know that you were 'meditating.' Mindfulness and meditation can come in many different forms, whether it's the act of meditating during a yoga session or if it's the act of simply being present in your life while folding the laundry. Mindfulness is a part of many different exercises and techniques to help people live a happier life.

There is, however, a basic form of mindfulness practice that you can use in any area of your life. We will look at some tips for how you can begin to practice this here, and you can then use this technique anytime you feel as though you are distracted or moving through your life on autopilot. You can even use it if you just need some time to be calm and in tune with your body and mind.

The most commonly practiced form of meditation is mindfulness meditation. This is also the most general type of meditation to help you facilitate mindfulness in all areas of your life. Mindfulness meditation is a type of mental training practice that involves you focusing your mind on your thoughts and sensations in the present moment (Agrawal, 2019). This includes your current emotions, physical sensations, and passing thoughts. Mindfulness meditation generally involves controlled breathing, mental imagery, self-awareness and muscle relaxation. It is typically easier for beginners to follow a guided meditation directing them throughout the whole process. It is extremely easy to drift away or fall asleep while in meditation if nobody is guiding you. Once you become more skilled in mindfulness meditation, you can do it without a vocal guide, but this requires strong mental capabilities.

Now, let's learn how you can practice mindfulness meditation. Most people do this for at least ten minutes each day. Even a couple minutes every single day can make a difference to your wellbeing. This is the basic technique that will help you get started:

1. Find a quiet place that you feel comfortable in—ideally, your home or someone where you feel safe. Sit in a chair or on the floor. Make sure your head and back are straight but are not tense.
2. Try to sort your thoughts and put aside those that are of the past and future. Stick to the thoughts about the present.
3. Bring your awareness to your breath. Make sure to focus on the feeling and sensation of air moving through your body as you inhale and exhale. Feel the way your belly rises and falls. Feel the air enter through your nostrils and leave through your mouth. Make sure to pay attention to the differences in each breath.
4. Watch every thought come and go. Act as if you are watching the clouds, letting them pass by you as you watch each one. Whether your thought is a worry, fear, anxiety, or hope - when these thoughts come up, don't ignore them or try to suppress them. Simply acknowledge them, remain calm, and anchor yourself with your breathing.
5. You may find yourself getting carried away in your thoughts. If this happens, observe where your mind went off to, and without making a judgment, simply return to your breathing. Keep in mind that this happens a lot with beginners; try not to be too hard on yourself when this happens. Always use your breathing as an anchor again.
6. As we near the end of the session, sit for a minute or two and become aware of where you physically are. Get up gradually.

You don't necessarily need to meditate to practice mindfulness. There are many other ways you can practice mindfulness without sitting down for a meditation session. However, I recommend you practice these methods when you are more experienced in mindfulness, as it will require much more focus and discipline.

Below are some examples of more specific scenarios in which you can practice mindfulness during your day. This will help you to reconnect with your inner self and with the environment around you.

- Doing the dishes

This is a great opportunity to practice meditation as typically nobody is trying to get your attention while you're doing the dishes. This perfect combination of alone time and physical activity makes a great window to try mindfulness.

Try to savor the feeling of the warm water on your hands. Savor the sensation and the appearance of the bubbles. Savor the smell of the dish soap, and the sound of pots and pans clunking under the water. If you're able to give yourself over to this experience, you'll end up with a refreshed mind and clean dishes!

- Brushing your teeth

Every single day you have to brush your teeth - this makes the normally boring task of dental hygiene a great opportunity to practice mindfulness.

Start by feeling your feet on the floor, the toothbrush in your hand, and the movement of your arm. Pay attention to this as you brush your teeth back and forth. A helpful tip is to pretend that there is a scanner - and that it is scanning your body from your feet up. Make sure to focus on the body part as the scanner moves from your feet to the top of your head.

- Driving

It is extremely easy for people to become mindless while driving. Especially if you're driving the same route day in and day out.

If you're driving to and from work, your mind typically wanders to what work tasks need to be completed that day, or the chores that you have to do once the day is over. Practice your mindfulness in the car as you're driving to keep yourself anchored inside the vehicle. Try to take in what's around you like the color of the car in front of you. The smell of the inside of your car. The way the steering wheel fits in your hands. Pay attention to all the noises you hear, from the music on the radio to the outside traffic noises. Whenever you find yourself wandering, bring your attention back to where you and your vehicle are in the moment.

- Exercising

Make your fitness routine an exercise in mindfulness by exercising away from screens and music. Focus on your breathing. Focus on where your feet are as you are moving. Sure, watching TV or listening to a podcast will make your run on the treadmill go by more quickly, but it won't do anything to quiet your mind. Allow yourself to feel the burn in your muscles and pay attention to how your body is reacting to the work out you are putting it through. Don't just ignore the pain of a muscle, acknowledge it, and let yourself feel the exercise.

- Bedtime

This is usually the time where you run around your home getting everything ready for your next long day, which is tomorrow. Don't battle too much with it; you know what needs to be done. Instead, stop trying to rush through it all and simply to try to enjoy the experience of doing the actual motions. Focus on the task at hand and don't think about the next task and the one after that. Leave yourself with enough time to not have to rush through the things you need to do. Again, any thoughts and anxieties that may come up this time, you may simply acknowledge them and let it pass.

- Mindful Eating

There are ways to eat which ensure that you are making the most of the time that you are eating, while also getting all of the nutrients that you need from your food. We will talk about something called mindful eating in more detail in the next section.

By paying attention to these important areas of your life and increasing your mindfulness in them, you can begin to see areas wherein which you can improve to help you live a happier life.

What Is Mindful Eating?

Mindful eating is when you really savor the moment, instead of being distracted by everything that is going on in your mind. Mindful eating is important as these are one of those tasks that we do numerous times per day. When we do a certain task repeatedly, our bodies will naturally try to automate that action to conserve energy.

However, when we eat mindlessly, we don't pay attention to the way food tastes, what we're eating, and how quickly we are consuming it. These bad automation habits are what causes us to mistreat our body. In this section, I will be teaching you the following:

- The basics of mindful eating
- How you can eat mindfully

- Exercises to help you practice this technique

The lack of mindful eating is something most of our population suffers from due to the increased pace of our lives. We typically find ourselves eating at work in front of our computer or eating dinner in front of the TV. Sometimes we may even eat during the commute to work! This seemingly small problem is actually one of the contributing factors in today's obesity and eating disorder problem. To combat this, we need to improve our ability to eat mindfully. Mindful eating uses the act of mindfulness to allow us to conquer common eating problems in our fast-paced lives (Beech, 2019).

The goal here is to shift focus from external thinking while eating, to joyfully delving into the eating experience itself. This is done to develop a new relationship with food. Here are a couple of points to help you identify when you are eating mindlessly.

- You are consistently eating until you are overly full or even feel sick
- You find yourself nibbling on food without really tasting it
- You aren't paying any attention to the foods you are eating and frequently eat in places that surround you with distractions
- You are rushing through your meals
- You have trouble remembering what you ate, or even the taste and smell of the last meal you've consumed

How Can Mindful Eating Benefit You?

- More Food Enjoyment in a Healthy Way

If you are feeling down emotionally when you do decide that it is time to eat, you may be focused on your emotional state and not really tasting or enjoying what you are eating. By practicing mindful eating, you will be present in your eating experience. This will help you to enjoy the taste of the food once again. It will also give you a chance to relax and relish in a few minutes of calm so that you can enjoy your food.

- Digestion

Ensuring that you eat mindfully comes with numerous benefits. One of these benefits is that it will help your body to digest more effectively. This will help you to get all the nutrients you need from your food.

- Decreases food cravings

Consciously eating will make you more aware of everything that you put into your mouth, and focusing on the experience of eating can help you to have fewer cravings and less desire to eat in between meals.

- Prevents overeating

This technique prevents overeating because you must pay attention to each bite that you put into your mouth. This will mean that you will be much more in tune with how full your body is.

- Improve your relationship with food

By using mindful eating, you will not be eating to make yourself feel better emotionally, but instead as nourishment for your precious body.

Practicing meditation is your first step in being able to achieve mindful eating. Allowing yourself to be mindful in your day to day life will bring new joys and satisfactions that have always been there but have not been noticed in some time, especially when it comes to a common activity like eating.

Steps Towards The Practice Of Mindful Eating

If you find yourself relating to the points I outlined in the first section; you may want to actively practice mindful eating. Follow these quick exercises below to begin increasing your level of mindfulness while eating.

- **Exercise #1: Prioritize your mealtimes.**

Try to isolate a 15-minute block to sit down and enjoy your meal. Don't eat on the go or skip meals because you're 'too busy.' Make sure you are always making time to eat at least three meals per day, no matter how busy you are.

- **Exercise #2: Avoid distractions while you are eating.**

It is impossible to enjoy eating your food when your attention is somewhere else. Try asking yourself how often you eat while in front of the TV, in the car, or in front of the computer. Eating under these circumstances is not mindful, and this can lead to overeating, choosing unhealthy options, or not enjoying the experience of your meal (Beech, 2019).

- **Exercise #3: Avoid being rushed around during meal times.**

Schedule a time block to eat your meal when you don't have any distractions around you. Even eating with a coworker or a friend may be a distraction due to conversation.

- **Exercise #4: Always sit down to eat your meal.**

When you go to eat, do so sitting down on a chair with your food on a table in front of you. This will help with digestion and help you to form a routine around eating. Try to avoid eating while standing up or walking as these create distractions. When you are physically up and about while eating, it will cause your mind to become distracted at the task at hand, as you will have to concentrate on your movement.

- **Exercise #5: Serve your meal on a plate or bowl.**

If possible, serve it on your favorite plate or bowl. Avoid eating food from the packet or take out containers as it makes eating feel less formal. This will help you pay more attention to your meal and its physical appearance.

- **Exercise #6: Make a conscious effort to chew your food thoroughly.**

Many people find themselves swallowing too soon and end up with digestion problems. Give your stomach an easier time with digesting by breaking down the food properly before swallowing.

- **Exercise #7: Make sure to eat only until you're 80% full.**

This is a fine line. Don't eat until you are certain you are full, but eat until you feel satisfied. A lot of the time, the feeling of fullness comes 10 minutes after you finish your meal. If you find yourself feeling full while you are still eating, you probably have overeaten.

- **Exercise #8: Take your time to truly savor the taste of food.**

Use all five of your senses. Before eating, take a look at your meal. Savor its look, smell, and overall appeal. Think about how each ingredient was cooked and seasoned and how you think the dish would taste because of it. During the meal, identify the taste of all the ingredients. What is the flavor? How does the flavor change if I eat different combinations of the ingredients? What can you smell? How does the texture feel in your mouth?

- **Exercise #9: Ask yourself how you feel about the food you are consuming.**

Do you feel happy? Pleasure? Guilt? Regret? Stress? Disappointment? Pay attention to the thoughts that the food brings to your mind. Does it bring up any memories? Fears? Beliefs? Give your food some serious consideration. How does your body feel after the meal compared to before? Do you feel energetic after eating, or do you feel lethargic? Does your stomach feel full or empty?

- **Exercise #10: Try to prepare your own meals where possible.**

The act of preparing food is proven to be psychologically beneficial and therapeutic. Make sure you are touching, tasting, and smelling the individual ingredients.

- **Exercise #11: Make a note of the difference in good food.**

This tends to be food that is fresh, seasonal, and minimally processed. Fresh and organic food tends to improve your overall mood and health. Food is our body's nourishment, and it provides the nutrition necessary for us to function optimally. Ingesting better quality food and ingredients is crucial to helping you feel better physically and psychologically.

How To Practice Mindful Eating

The key to mindful eating is to use all five of your senses. Doing this will bring your consciousness and your state of awareness into the present moment. This will also help you to avoid distractions. To practice mindful eating, try following along with the exercise below during your next meal, and try to do so every meal after that. Eventually, you will be able to practice this every time you eat.

Before you take a bite of your food, notice the smells of the food you are about to eat. Notice how it looks- the colors and textures. As you put food in your mouth, feel the textures of the food on your tongue. Notice all of the flavors that you are tasting and the feeling that they bring to your mouth. Notice how it feels when you chew the food- how it feels on your teeth and your cheeks. Doing this with every bite will bring you into the moment and ensure that you are consciously eating. Try practicing this with every meal.

Chapter 7: Intuitive Eating Meal Planning

Once you have come up with your general plan for your new lifestyle and how you want it to look, you can then begin planning more specifically. After you have gained an understanding of the principles of intuitive eating, you will be well equipped to begin this new style of eating.

What Is Meal Planning?

Planning your individual meals will make it much easier for you to reach for something nutritious and delicious when you are short on time. For example, when you get home from work or when you wake up tired in the morning and need to pack something for your lunch, you will not need to spend time planning your meals for the day.

You can plan your meals out a week in advance, two weeks or even a month if you wish. You can post this up on your fridge, and each day you will know exactly what you have ready to go, with no thinking required. When you do this, you will be able to step up to your fridge at dinner time and choose something that you want to eat you know you will provide your body with the nutrients it needs. You can heat it up in the oven and then begin to eat mindfully at the table.

By doing this preparation and planning in advance, you will allow yourself to benefit from eating healthy food and also the right proportion of food. Since you will have already planned out your meals, as well as each portion, you will take out the thinking, which will leave space for you to practice your mindful eating.

How Does Meal Planning Differ With Intuitive Eating Versus Dieting?

Regular meal planning involves looking at the week ahead and planning what you are going to eat based on the diet that you are following. For example, if you are on a Ketogenic diet, you would plan your meals with high-fat content and low carbohydrate content, and you would eat these meals during the week, regardless of what you feel like eating.

With intuitive meal planning, you will be able to plan your eating and thus, provide yourself with quick and easy meals that you can reheat or place in the oven in a pinch. This does not mean that you will stick to any specific diet plan. Rather, you will follow your intuitive eating principles to eat according to your body's signals. Having food prepared in advance will allow you to have fresh and healthy meals readily available to nourish your body. When you become hungry, you have healthy food right at your fingertips.

How To Meal Plan With Intuitive Eating

When it comes to meal planning with intuitive eating, you want to pre-prepare meals that will allow you to enjoy healthy and delicious options whenever you feel hungry. For this reason, you do not need to prepare specific meals to eat at specific times, but rather meals that you can reach for whenever you need them, knowing that you will enjoy the food. These meals will also be meals that you know will provide your body with the essential nutrients that it needs.

You can also prepare healthy snacks and treats that are actually good for you. There is nothing more rewarding than making your brain feel nourished while also replenishing your body. This can be as simple as a homemade trail mix with a bit of dark chocolate or a proportioned smoothie mix.

When you prepare food to eat for the week, try and add your favorite flavors to healthy food, and don't forget to keep it exciting with variety!

Chapter 8: Intuitive Eating Recipes

In this chapter, I will share with you some delicious recipes that you can try at home. These recipes are great for those who wish to try something new in the kitchen or who are becoming bored with their regular cycle of dinner meals.

Intuitive Eating Recipe Examples

Below are several recipes that you can try to make on your own at home so that you can feed your body new and delicious meals anytime!

Delicious Coconut Date Smoothie

Preparation Time: 5 Minutes
Cook Time: 1 Minute
Total Time: 6 Minutes

Ingredients:
- 2 cups almond milk or coconut milk
- 4 dates, (pitted)
- ¼ Cup spinach, frozen
- ¼ Cup chard, frozen (if possible)
- ¼ Cup kale, frozen (if possible)
- 1 cup strawberries, frozen
- 2 bananas
- 1 tbsp Chia seeds

- A small handful of ice cubes. You can adjust this amount depending on how many of your ingredients are frozen and how thick you want your smoothie to be.

Instructions
1. In your blender, add the almond milk, the dates, the spinach, kale, and the chard. We begin with only these

ingredients as they require extra blending because of all of their surface area.
2. Now, add in the strawberries, the two bananas, and the amount of ice that you have chosen. Blend until smooth
3. Pour into a large cup and add the chia seeds on top.
4. Serve and eat with a spoon or a straw

Egg And Avocado Rice Bowl

The first recipe we will look at is an Egg and Avocado Brown Rice Bowl. This recipe uses brown rice, garlic, and avocado, which are all good sources of Vitamin B6 or Pyridoxine. If you are a vegetarian, you can leave out the salmon, but if you add it, then you will be getting vitamin B1, or thiamine, as well as Omega-3 fatty acids. Further, the broccoli contains folic acid, and so does avocado. The egg used is also one that has been fortified with Omega-3.

Preparation Time: 10 Minutes
Cook Time: 40 Minutes
Total Time: 50 Minutes
Serves: 1

Ingredients:
- 1 Omega-3 Egg
- ¼ cup thinly sliced green onion
- Small bunch of broccoli
- Extra Virgin Olive Oil
- Half Avocado, sliced
- 1 Tsp Sesame Seeds
- 1 Tsp pickled ginger
- 1 Cup brown rice
- Salt and Pepper
- Splash Rice Wine Vinegar
- 1 salmon fillet

Instructions:
1. Bring your salmon out from the fridge so that it will be room temperature when you are ready to cook it.
2. Cook your brown rice according to its instructions. Feel free to make extra if you wish to expand this recipe into multiple portions or to save some for later to reheat.

3. If you are cooking the rice on the stovetop and you are unsure how you can follow the following instructions;
4. Put 1 cup of rinsed brown rice in a pot with 1 teaspoon of olive oil and 2 cups of water.
Bring the pot to a boil, then cover it and reduce the heat to low.
Simmer this pot of rice, water, and olive oil for 45 minutes.
Remove the rice from the burner and leave it to sit with its cover still on for approximately 10 minutes.
Fluff your rice with a fork to give it that loose texture.
5. With about twenty minutes left on your rice, preheat your oven to 400 degrees Fahrenheit. Cut your broccoli florets into small bite-size pieces and prepare your broccoli for roasting by placing the florets on a baking sheet and drizzle them with some olive oil. Sprinkle salt and pepper to taste. Toss them to spread the olive oil and the salt and pepper evenly. Place the baking sheet in the oven when it is preheated. Roast them in the oven until they are browned, and the stems are softened about fifteen minutes.
6. To cook your salmon, warm a non-stick pan on medium to low heat and place some drizzles of olive oil into the pan. Season your salmon as you wish with salt and pepper and then place it in the pan with the skin facing up. Cook for about four minutes, or until it is golden brown, and then flip it. On this second side, cook it until it is firm when you press into it, and the skin becomes crispy. This second side will take roughly three minutes.
7. When your rice and your broccoli is almost finished, fry your egg in a pan with a bit of olive oil until it is cooked through.
8. You can either remove the skin from your salmon or leave it on, whichever you wish.
9. When your broccoli is ready, place it on your rice bowl along with your salmon. Then add your fried egg, your sliced

avocado, your sliced green onion, pickled ginger, and finally, the sesame seeds. Add a splash of rice wine vinegar to the bowl and you are ready to eat.

Breakfast Oats

A great breakfast recipe and one that you can prepare in a very short amount of time. Whole grain oats contain iron, and if you add fruits to it like bananas and raspberries, these contain magnesium. The apricots will give the oats sweetness without sugar and also contain iron. Adding nuts like almonds will give you protein and adding milk or yogurt as well will add calcium to your diet.

Preparation Time: 5 Minutes
Cook Time: 5 Minutes
Total time: 5 Minutes

Serves 1
Ingredients:
- ¾ Cup plain Whole grain oats
- ¼ cup almonds, sliced
- ½ Banana, sliced
- ¼ Cup raspberries
- ¾ Cup cinnamon, ground
- ¼ Cup dried apricots

Instructions:
1. Add the oats and 1 ½ cups of water to a small pot. Turn on the burner to high heat and bring these ingredients up to a boil. When this occurs, turn the heat down to medium to low and let it cook for five minutes, or until there is no water left unabsorbed.
2. Remove this from the heat and then transfer the cooked oats to a bowl.
3. Pour in the cinnamon, the almonds, bananas, apricots, and raspberries in whatever order you wish.
4. Eat it while still hot for best taste

Braised Chicken On A Bed Of Lentils And Mushrooms

This recipe contains chicken thighs which are an excellent source of vitamin K2, as well as lentils which will provide you with your calcium and mushrooms which are the only plant source that naturally contains Vitamin D. This recipe is a triple threat when it comes to your health, and it tastes great to boot!

Preparation Time: 10 Minutes
Cook Time: 35 Minutes
Total Time: 45 Minutes

Serves 4
Ingredients:

- 4 chicken thighs
- 1 onion
- 2 Cups Mushrooms of your choice (400g)
- 2 Cups lentils (green or any of your choice)
- 2 cloves of garlic, diced
- 2 Tbsp olive oil
- 2.5 cups water
- 1 tsp salt
- Black pepper grinder
- ⅔ Cup chicken broth (low sodium)
- 2 tbsp parsley, chopped
- 2 tbsp lemon juice

Instructions:
1. In a large pot, add the lentils and the water as well as ¾ of the tsp of salt. Bring this to a boil on high heat.
2. Once boiling, bring the heat down to low to medium heat and let the lentils simmer with a lid covering the pot for 25 minutes. You want the lentils to be soft but not breaking into pieces.

3. While the lentils are cooking, get a large pan and place 1 tbsp of olive oil in it. Add the onion, the garlic, and the mushrooms. Cook this on low heat until the onions turn clear and are aromatic.
4. When the lentils are done, add the mixture of onions, garlic, and mushrooms to the lentils in the pot.
5. Add 1 tbsp of oil in the now-empty pan on medium heat.
6. While you are doing this, use ¼ teaspoon of salt and some black pepper and put the chicken into the heated pan.
7. Cook the chicken until it becomes browned. This will take roughly 12 minutes.
8. Pour the remaining oil and any fat out of the pan and into a small bowl. Don't throw this out yet.
9. Add your chicken broth to the pan with chicken and then bring the heat down to low and put a lid on the pan before letting it simmer for 15 minutes.
10. Add the juice and fat that you put aside earlier to the pit of lentils and vegetables.
11. Add as well the chopped parsley and some lemon juice to the pot of lentils and vegetables.
12. Add the now cooked chicken into the lentils pot and put the lid on. Let this sit for 5 minutes.
13. After the 5 minutes have passed, you are ready to eat!
14. Garnish with salt and pepper if you wish, plate, and serve.

Beef And Broccoli Stir-Fry

Preparation Time: 16 minutes
Cooking time: 12 minutes
Total Time: 28 minutes

Makes: 4 Servings
Serving Size: 1 and ¼ of a cup or ¼ of total recipe

Ingredients:
- Sirloin Beef, Lean and thinly sliced- ¾ of a pound
- Cornstarch- 2 and 1/3 tablespoons
- Red pepper flakes- 2 tablespoons
- Chicken Broth, Reduced Sodium- 1 Cup
- Salt- ¼ teaspoon
- Broccoli- 5 cups
- Water- ¼ cup
- Ginger root, minced- 1 tablespoon
- Garlic, minced- 2 tablespoons
- Soy Sauce, low sodium- ¼ cup

Instructions:
1. Take a large plate and spread the cornstarch and the salt around the plate evenly. Take the beef strips and coat them with the mixture.
2. Using a wok or a deep pan, put the oil in and heat it up on the medium to high heat level
3. Put the beef in when the pan is hot and cook this until it is cooked all the way through- you will know as it will turn brown. This will take about 4 minutes.
4. Use a slotted spoon and take the beef out of the pan and place it on a new plate.
5. In the same pan with the heated oil and the beef drippings, put ½ cup of reduced-sodium chicken broth. Begin stirring this in the pan to combine everything and loosen the residue on the pan.

6. Put the broccoli in the pan and cook it with the lid on. Add some water if you need it.
7. When the broccoli is becoming softer but not fully cooked yet- this will take about 3 minutes, take the lid off and put the garlic, ginger, and red pepper flakes in. Fry this until it becomes noticeably fragrant, which will take roughly one minute.
8. Using a vessel of your choice, mix the rest of the broth (1/2 cup), the soy sauce, the water, and the rest of the cornstarch (1/2 tablespoon). Stir it to mix well.
9. Put this sauce mix into the wok and stir everything to combine it all.
10. Bring the heat down to a medium to low level and let this simmer.
11. Simmer for about a minute, until it begins to become thicker.
12. Put the beef in the pan once again and stir everything, so the beef becomes coated.
13. It is now ready to serve!

Intuitive Eating With Food Allergies Or Restrictions

You may be wondering, at this point in the book, what you should do, or if it is even possible for you to practice intuitive eating if you have allergies or food restrictions. The answer to this question is a resounding "Yes". No matter your allergies or dietary restrictions, it is possible to practice intuitive eating.

Since intuitive eating aims to help you get back to your body's natural state of being, where you follow its desires and needs, you can practice this no matter what foods you normally eat. Whether you are a vegetarian, a vegan, have celiac disease, are allergic to peanuts or anything else, you can still listen to your body, follow the nine rules of intuitive eating and get back to your body's preferred method of eating.

Tips For Intuitive Eating With Food Allergies Or Restrictions

- Listen to your body

While you cannot give in to every craving or every desire that your body has, you can still listen to your body when it comes to intuitive eating with allergies or dietary restrictions. You can listen to when your body is hungry, what your body needs to eat or drink, or how much it needs to eat.

- Adhere to your restrictions or allergies

Just because you are practicing intuitive eating does not mean that you need to give into every type of food item that you feel like eating. You can still maintain your prescribed diet while practicing intuitive eating, while avoiding the foods you are allergic to. As long as you keep this in mind, all of the other rules of intuitive eating still apply.

Intuitive Eating Recipes For Food Allergies Or Restrictions

Below you can find recipes that will help you to make delicious and healthy foods while still adhering to your dietary restrictions or allergies.

Fresh Green Beans with Tofu And Mushroom Stir-Fry

If you are a vegetarian, this recipe is a great option for a quick and delicious dinner that does not include meat, and that instead includes tofu as a great protein source.

Nutritional Information:
Serving: 1 Serving (1/6 of Recipe)
Calories: 94kcal
Carbohydrates: 9g
Protein: 5g
Fat: 5g
Saturated Fat: 2g
Fiber: 3g
Sugar: 4g

15 minutes: Prep Time
20 minutes: Cook Time
35 minutes: Total Time

Servings: 6 Servings

Ingredients:
- 1/4 teaspoon kosher salt
- 1-pound thin green beans trimmed
- 1 cup tofu, firm variety
- 1 tablespoon minced fresh sage
- 1 large shallot minced
- 12 ounces mushrooms thinly sliced

- 1 teaspoon olive oil
- 3 tablespoons parsley minced
- 1 tablespoon minced fresh thyme leaves
- 1/4 teaspoon freshly ground black pepper
- 1 tablespoon ginger, grated
- 1 tablespoon soy sauce

Instructions:
1. Salt a large saucepan full of water and heat it up until it boils. Mix your beans into the water and cook them until they become tender but still a little crispy, this will take approximately 2 minutes. Drain the water and immediately move the cooked beans to a bowl full of ice and water to stop them from cooking any further.
2. Drain the beans of the water once again and set them aside.
3. Put your tofu inside of a big frying pan on one-half level of heat. Heat your tofu until it becomes crispy. Move the tofu to a paper towel and crumble it with your hands before setting it off to the side for later.
4. Put olive oil into the same frying pan you used before and turn it on to medium-high heat. Add in your mushrooms and shallots, and cook them until they are tender, this will take approx—2 to 3 minutes.
5. Add the green beans to the frying pan again and cook the entire thing for 1 to 2 minutes more, stir it often.
6. Add in the sage, thyme, parsley, pepper and, salt, and stir it to combine. Cook this for another minute, before re-adding your tofu.
7. Serve this dish either hot or at room temperature.

Vegan Chana Masala Curry

If you are vegan, this is a delicious and healthy curry recipe that you can make that also adheres to your diet restrictions.

Nutritional Information:
Calories: 371
Calories from Fat: 88
Total Fat: 10g
Carbohydrates: 59 grams
Protein: 17 grams

Servings: Makes 4 Servings

Ingredients:
- Olive Oil- 1 Tablespoon
- Cayenne Pepper- 1/8 of a tablespoon
- Diced Tomatoes- 28 ounces diced
- Garam Masala- 2 tablespoons
- Jalapeno Pepper- 1
- Onion- 1 diced
- Ginger- 1 tablespoon shaved
- Garlic- 4 cloves minced
- Chickpeas- canned- 28 ounces (be sure to drain the liquid and rinse them before using them in the recipe)

Instructions:
1. Take a big wok and put the olive oil into it
2. Once heated, add in your onions and sauté them until they are sweating and softened. This will take about 5 minutes.
3. Add in your ginger, jalapeno, and your garlic, and then cook this mixture for another minute
4. Sprinkle in your spices (pepper, salt, coriander, turmeric, garam masala, cumin, cayenne pepper). Then, cook this for another minute. The mixture will become fragrant as you do this.
5. Add your chickpeas and tomatoes into the fragrant mixture in the wok. Let this simmer.

6. Cover the pan and let this simmer for about twenty minutes.
7. After it simmers for the allotted time, give it a taste test and season it if you feel it could be spicier or if it needs more salt. You might want to mix in some more of the garam masala if you want it to be stronger in flavor.
8. Serve and enjoy this meal that is only 1 Smart Point per serving!

Chapter 9: Intuitive Eating While Pregnant

You may have heard of the whacky cravings that many women experience during pregnancy. With the onset of the second trimester come these very strong cravings that nobody can truly understand but the pregnant woman who is needing ice cream with pickles right away! The second trimester is when these cravings will be at an all-time high. You may also experience some aversions to certain foods at the same time as your cravings begin around the end of the first and beginning of the second trimester.

You may wonder "when it is okay to give in to these cravings"? Some of them may be for things that are not wildly unhealthy, like a sandwich with lots of mustard or some sweet things like fruits mixed in with pudding. These cravings are okay to give in to from time to time, especially if they are fleeting. You must ensure, however, that the majority of your meals are balanced and healthy, giving both you and your baby the nutrients you need.

Craving Examples And Substitutions

- Carbohydrates

If you crave foods like carbohydrates, try to combine them with a protein. An example of this is cheese and crackers. This is a healthier snack than crackers alone.

- Fast Foods

If you are feeling a lot of cravings that are for candies, chips, fast-foods and other objectively unhealthy foods most of the time, it will not be beneficial to you and your baby to eat these foods every day. Supplements can sometimes help with a situation like this, where you will be craving certain foods and unable to stomach others. Supplements can help you to get the vitamins and nutrients that you need if you cannot get them from real foods. Your first option, however, should always be natural food.

- Caffeine

Another craving that will likely be nagging at you during the beginning of your pregnancy is the craving for caffeine. It is always important to watch your caffeine intake during pregnancy.

Caffeine is okay in very small amounts, but it should not be consumed at high levels. This is especially important in the first trimester because of the potential of miscarriage that it can cause. Caffeine consumption during pregnancy has also been shown to lead to premature delivery as well as low birth weight. In some cases, a baby can even exhibit withdrawal symptoms from caffeine. To be safe, it is better to avoid caffeine, especially in the first trimester.

Caffeine also dehydrates the consumer, so it is essential to ensure you are properly hydrated if you are consuming any caffeine. Instead of coffee, try drinking an herbal tea or flavored water to give yourself a pleasant drink to sip on.

Foods To Avoid

While you can certainly follow intuitive eating during pregnancy, some foods should be avoided when pregnant. Though intuitive eating does not involve any kind of restriction or diet mentality, it is important to ensure that you are keeping both yourself and your baby safe. In this section, we will look at the foods that you should not eat while pregnant.

- Listeria

Deli meats can sometimes contain Listeria, which is a bacteria that is not as serious to adults on our own, but if you are pregnant, this can be very damaging to your unborn baby. The reason why listeria is so damaging is that it can reach the baby through the placenta and can poison the baby's blood or give it an infection, which could potentially lead to a miscarriage.

Smoked Foods should be avoided for the same reason as deli meats, as these can contain listeria as well. These foods include smoked fish, (like lox) as well as meat jerky.

Soft Cheeses like blue cheese, feta, and queso should be avoided because they can also contain listeria. The unpasteurized milk used to make this cheese is what makes them potentially harmful. Though, if the soft cheese is not imported, and if it is made with pasteurized milk, it is likely safe.

- Tuna

While tuna doesn't need to be avoided altogether, canned tuna should be consumed at a minimum as well as other fish such as mackerel and swordfish. These types of fish are known to contain mercury at higher levels than others. Mercury can be harmful to your baby by causing brain development issues or brain damage, so be sure to avoid these. Especially during the first trimester when everything in the baby's body is rapidly forming. Be careful when eating sushi as sometimes the fish used in sushi can contain mercury in high amounts.

- Salmonella

Salmonella is harmful to humans if they become infected, but it is even more harmful to unborn babies. Salmonella can infect the fluid that surrounds the baby in the placenta, which can then lead to a miscarriage. Salmonella poisoning can cause the mother to become quite sick, which is not ideal for a woman who is carrying a growing baby. This is because all of her resources need to go towards helping the baby to grow into a strong and healthy individual.

To avoid risking exposure to salmonella, **raw eggs,** and anything containing raw eggs should be avoided altogether. Some dressings and sauces can contain raw eggs, and so you should be careful when consuming these. Further, **raw meats** can contain salmonellae such as chicken, turkey, **raw seafood,** and rare beef such as steaks.

Avoid eating uncooked clams, oysters, eggs, and meats like a rare steak. This can leave you at risk of different foodborne pathogens that can harm your baby.

In the third trimester, you should avoid the same things as you should avoid in the first and second trimesters like smoked fish and meats, deli meats, uncooked eggs, raw meats, and caffeine. There are some additional things to avoid as well in this trimester, though, which are listed below for you.

- Cat litter

You should avoid cat litter as it can contain a parasite that has been known to lead to toxoplasmosis. This can also be contracted through **undercooked meat**. This disease can be transmitted to your baby if you are infected with it, which is why it should be heavily prevented. This disease can give flu-like symptoms, which to an adult may not be so bad, but to an unborn baby, this could be detrimental.

- Uncooked sprouts

Uncooked sprouts should also be avoided. Bacteria like those we discussed in the previous chapters- listeria and salmonella in addition to E.coli, can be found in sprouts because of the cracks in their shells. So, if you want to eat them, you must thoroughly cook them first to kill any bacteria that maybe there.

- Raw fish

Raw fish should be avoided. This is because it contains mercury, which is unhealthy for your unborn baby. Cooked fish are safe to eat, but only eeaten in moderate quantities- no more than twice per week.

Intuitive Eating Post-Pregnancy

After giving birth, it is important to take some time to rest and recuperate. Beginning a strict diet immediately after giving birth in an attempt to lose extra weight, is not a good idea. This is because a weight loss diet will reduce the quality of breast milk that your body produces.

Believe it or not, performing the act of breastfeeding each day causes you to burn calories. Just like when you were still pregnant, you will still need to consume more calories than you regularly would have before you became pregnant. For this reason, don't go on any sort of diet while breastfeeding, and don't begin to watch what you eat unless it is to ensure you are eating enough of the nutrients that you and your baby need. You will want to have as many nutrients and calories as your baby requires, so listen to your hunger and follow what it is telling you, especially while breastfeeding.

Caffeine Post-Pregnancy

If you were a regular coffee drinker before you became pregnant, you will likely be looking for the coffee pot after giving birth.

The problem is, it is important to watch your caffeine consumption while breastfeeding. Caffeine has been shown to affect breastmilk, and therefore, the baby as well. Having too much caffeine as a breastfeeding mother can lead to your baby receiving it through the milk and, in turn, becoming fussy and extra energetic afterward. You also want to avoid having your baby become dependent on caffeine, as this is not healthy. Caffeine can also lead to dehydration, and the last thing you want is a dehydrated baby. You can have some caffeine, but no more than 24 ounces per day, preferably in 3 different 8-ounce servings and no more than this.

Bonus: How to Teach Your Child Mindful Eating

Since our childhood and developmental history play a big role in who we are today, it is important to raise your child in an intentional way, instilling habits and beliefs that will benefit them early on. In this chapter, we will look at how you can raise a mindful eater and a child who practices intuitive eating.

How To Transform Your Child's Relationship With Food

In this section, we are going to discuss several ways that you can help your child to develop a healthy relationship with food.

- Avoid using food as a reward

If you teach your child that food is used as a reward, it can lead them away from intuitive eating and towards an unhealthy relationship with food.

- Avoid using food as a punishment

Similar to how using food as a reward can lead your child to develop an unhealthy relationship with food, using food as a punishment t can lead your child to develop an unhealthy relationship with food. Examples of this include withholding food or not allowing certain foods as a form of punishment.

- Set a good example

Food can be seen as something that you need to survive, as a form of stress-relief through the enjoyment of cooking healthy foods and as a way to bring people together. By viewing food and food preparation in this way, you can shift your perspective and change your relationship with food. By doing this within your own life, you can impart this wisdom on your child and help them develop into a little human with a healthy relationship to food.

How To Encourage Your Child To Practice Intuitive Eating

To help your child become an intuitive eater, one of the greatest things that you can do is model this type of behavior for them. Using the information in this chapter, you will be able to help your child have a better relationship with food. This will also help you to develop your child into an intuitive eater.

For the most part, children are already much better equipped to become successful intuitive eaters, as they have not been exposed to the diet culture and all of the shame and punishment that comes with it. For this reason, teaching them about intuitive eating will likely be much easier and require much less work than teaching yourself or other adults.

Children are usually better able to practice mindfulness than adults can, as they are likely get in touch with the sensations and feelings of their body with much more ease than adults can. By encouraging them and reminding them that they should listen to their body, they will not be as affected by the media and the diet culture that will eventually make its way into their view.

How To Encourage Your Child To Practice Mindful Eating

We have discussed mindfulness several times throughout this book, and here we are going to discuss how you can encourage your child to become a mindful eater.

Mindfulness is not a practice that is reserved only for adults; mindfulness is a technique that can be performed by children as well. Mindfulness can help children to fine-tune their mind-body connection. One great way to do this is to help your child perform the body scan meditation, as you learned in the "listen to your body" section of this book. This practice will help them to identify what they are feeling physically and mentally, and where they are feeling it as well. By helping your child to practice this kind of mindfulness, you will introduce them to the idea of mindfulness, and you can then incorporate it into their eating practices. Once you get them acquainted with their bodies from the inside out, doing this while sitting at the table for a meal will be much easier for them.

Further, scientific research points to the conclusion that there are numerous physical and psychological benefits to relieving tension and relaxing your body, even for children. The body scan meditation is a very effective and useful meditation technique that can help both you and your child to stay physically and mentally relaxed. It can help you return to a calm state when you notice that your child is not being mindful at the dinner table. This could be caused by a large number of distractions, for example. Here is a guide on how you can try the body scan meditation. You may wish to try this on your own first, and then try it with your child by reading out the directions to them and helping them if they have any questions.

In no time, your child will be able to do an abbreviated version of this meditation by sitting down and bringing awareness to any place in your body where you feel that you are carrying tension. This can then translate to the dinner table, where they can bring attention and awareness to their mouth and eating food.

Another great way to help your child practice mindfulness is by walking them through a basic mindfulness meditation that is great for beginners. Begin by reading the following instructions aloud to them in a low and soft voice, encouraging relaxation and attention to their body. Remind them of the benefits that mindful eating can provide them with, such as better digestion, better relaxation, and overall healthier eating habits.

1. Find a quiet place that you feel comfortable in—ideally, your home or someone where you feel safe. Sit in a chair or on the floor. Make sure your head and back are straight but are not tense.
2. Try to sort your thoughts and put aside those that are of the past and future. Stick to the thoughts about the present.
3. Bring your awareness to your breath. Make sure to focus on the feeling and sensation of air moving through your body as you inhale and exhale. Feel the way your belly rises and falls. Feel the air enter through your nostrils and leave through your mouth. Make sure to pay attention to the differences in each breath.
4. Watch every thought come and go. Act as if you are watching the clouds, letting them pass by you as you watch each one. Whether your thought is a worry, fear, anxiety, or hope - when these thoughts come up, don't ignore them or try to suppress them. Simply acknowledge them, remain calm, and anchor yourself with your breathing.
5. You may find yourself getting carried away in your thoughts. If this happens, observe where your mind wandered, and without passing judgment on yourself, return focus to your breaths. Keep in mind that this happens a lot with beginners; try not to be too hard on yourself when this occurs. Always use your breathing as an anchor again.
6. As we near the end of the session, sit for a minute or two and become aware of where you physically are. Get up gradually.

By helping your child to practice this type of mindfulness meditation, you will be able to encourage them to use this practice when they are at the dinner table. Eventually, your entire family will be able to practice mindful eating at the table together and experience the joys that intuitive eating can bring to your life.

Intuitive Eating Quick Tips

Before this book concludes, I want to leave you with a few more tips to stay on course with intuitive eating.

- Tip 1: Self-Evaluate

Before you begin, take some time to look at your existing eating habits, patterns, and behaviors and analyze them.

- Tip 2: Self-Rank

When you finish eating a meal, rank your level of fullness on a scale of 1 to 10, 1 being extremely hungry and 10 being extremely stuffed. This will help you to determine if you are successfully stopping when you are satisfied and not overeating.

- Tip 3: Listen

As you know by now, listening to your body, your emotions and your mind is extremely important when it comes to intuitive eating. As long as you remember this, you will be well on your way to becoming a lifelong intuitive eater.

- Tip 4: Keep Practicing

If you have learned anything in this book, it is that you should allow yourself the space to learn and grow. Making mistakes is part of the journey. You should allow yourself to learn as you go and do not expect perfection right away. If you are dedicated to becoming an intuitive eater, you should allow yourself the time to practice. Just like any skill, you will need to practice and develop your skills of listening to your body and giving it what it needs.

- Tip 5: Maintain a "Growth Mindset"

Success depends on whether or not a person has a growth mindset. A fixed mindset is when a person believes that their intelligence and skills are a fixed trait (O'Brien 2018). They have what they have, and that's it. This makes the person highly concerned with what skills and intelligence they currently have, and they do not focus on what they can gain. Therefore, their activities are limited to the capacity that they think they have. However, those with growth mindsets understand that any skill can be developed and improved upon throughout their life.

This can be done through education, training, or simply just even passion. They understand that their brain is a muscle that can be 'worked out' to grow stronger. Knowing this, you must employ a growth mindset. Every single skill you have can be ameliorated by putting in the effort to see it from a growth mindset. This is the mindset for success when it comes to life in general, but especially when it comes to changing something about your lifestyle- like learning to practice intuitive eating.

Conclusion

You began this book as someone who was unable to stop disordered overeating and who was unsure of where to turn for support and advice. Now, you have found the solution to this problem and have learned everything you need to know about the "non-diet method of intuitive eating." In this book, we discussed intuitive eating and intuitive movement at-length. Now you are equipped with a solution once and for all! This method has been proven to work for many people. You are now ready to put this into practice, where you will find yourself with a new lease on life.

In this book, we discussed what intuitive eating is and the science behind why it works. We also discussed the benefits that you will find through following an intuitive eating style, and we looked at the nine rules of intuitive eating, which include the following:

1. Adhere to your hunger
2. Say no to the diet industry
3. Don't restrict what you eat
4. Recognize when you are full
5. Eliminate dietary thinking
6. Don't eat out of "emotional hunger."
7. Don't self-judge
8. Exercise using intuitive movement
9. Listen to your body

In addition to these principles, we also looked at what emotional eating is and how you can make peace with your body. You learned how to properly compose your plate of food, develop a meal plan and engage in mindful eating. You were also given several nutritious recipes that you can try at home.

Finally, we looked at some tips for intuitive eating for women who are pregnant and for parents who wish to raise their children as mindful eaters. All of these topics and more made for a book packed with valuable information that will be available to you any time you need it.

As you begin your journey of intuitive eating, you will find that you develop a higher level of self-esteem, along with, better feelings about your body image. You find that you have more optimism about life in general. You also have numerous health benefits including a lower body mass index, higher HDL cholesterol levels and lower triglyceride levels. Emotional and disordered eating finally becomes less frequent. With all this being said, you are well on your way to becoming the best version of yourself.

The one major takeaway that I want you to get through reading this book is a new perspective on dieting and eating well. I also want you to walk away with a new perspective on exercise and movement of your body. With these new ways of viewing your body and yourself, I want you to leave this book with a new sense of self and a new lease on life. You have taken your health into your own hands, and you are now able to see that you don't have to force yourself to follow a diet that is doomed from the start or an exercise plan that does not fit with your body or your mind. If you can understand this, you have gained the most valuable piece of information that this book has to offer you. Today is the best today to start improving your health. Good luck on your journey!

References

"Body Scan Meditation" (2019, April 16). Retrieved from https://www.igrc.org/blogpostsdetail/body-scan-meditation-12794843

Agrawal, A. (2019, June 20). *Mindfulness Meditation – What It Is And How To Do It*. Inspired Journey towards greater heights -learnings and sharing. Retrieved from https://befinexpert.wordpress.com/2019/06/20/mindfulness-meditation-what-it-is-and-how-to-do-it

Beech, S. (2019). *Mindful Eating*. The Psych Professionals. Retrieved from https://psychprofessionals.com.au/mindful-eating

O'Brien, D. (2018, August 1). *Back to School With a Growth Mindset*. Dynamath. Retrieved from https://dynamath.scholastic.com/pages/dynamath-expressions/2018-19/back-to-school-with-a-growth-mindset.html

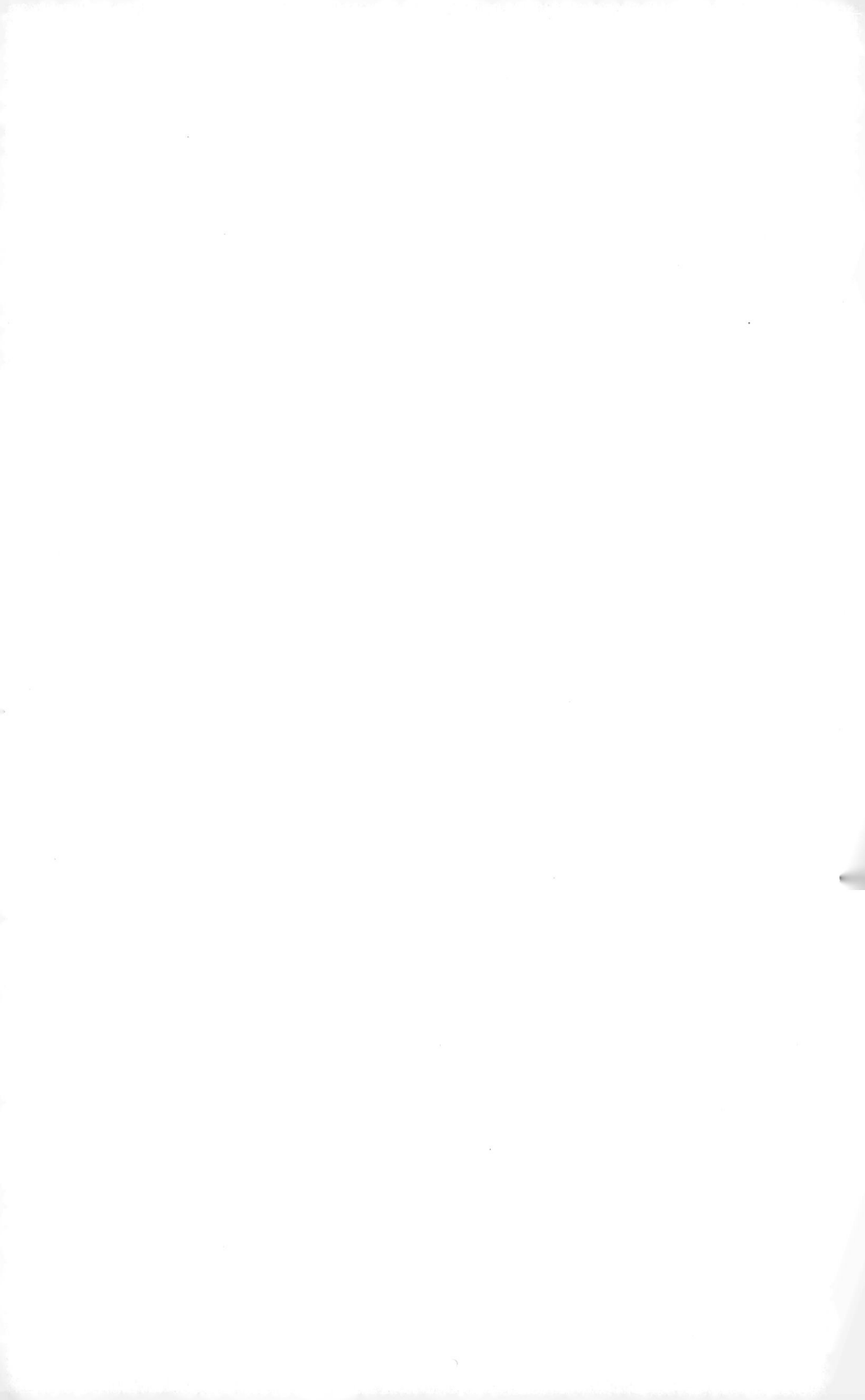

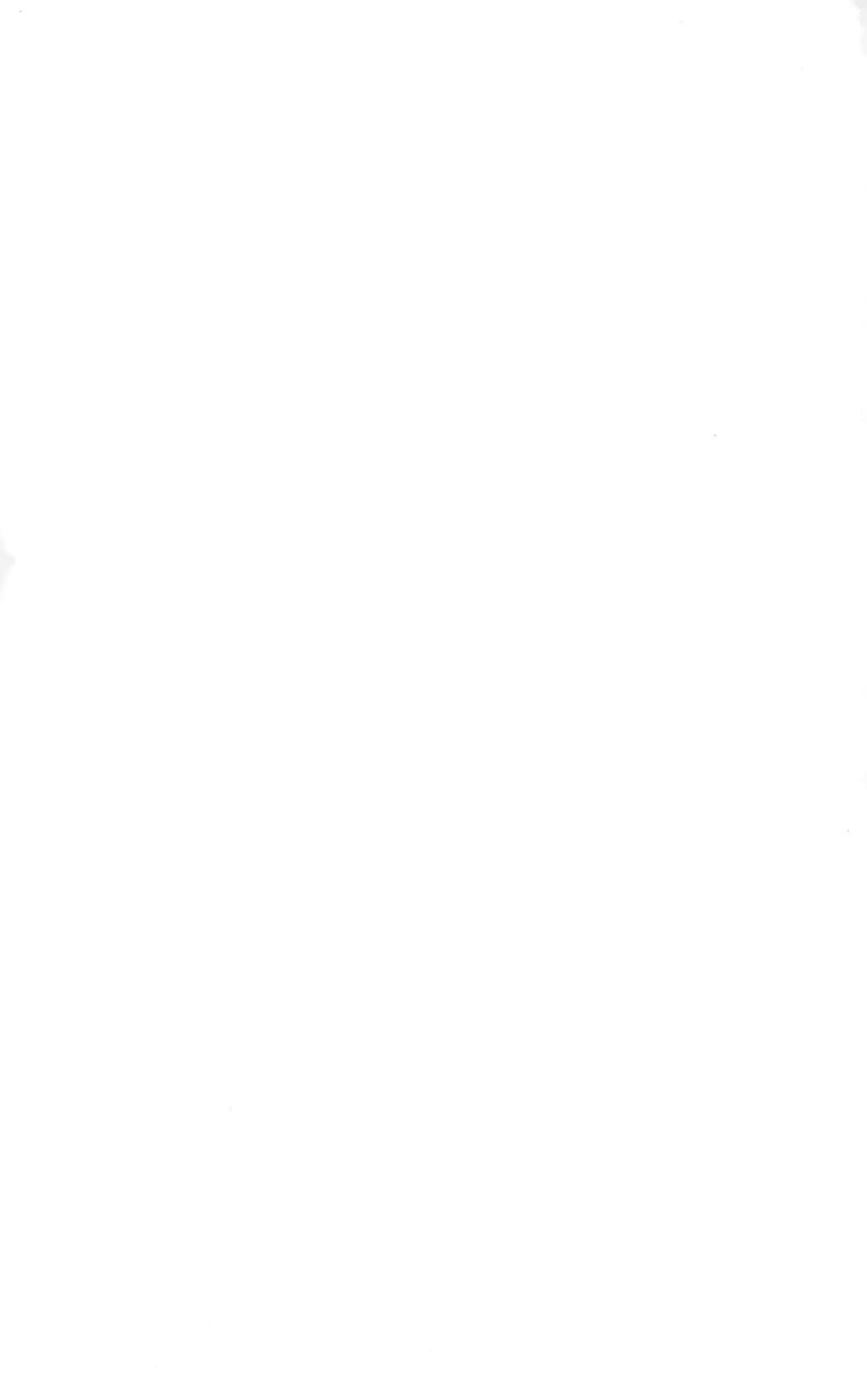

Printed in Great Britain
by Amazon